AF574115

MAINSTREAMS OF MEDICINE

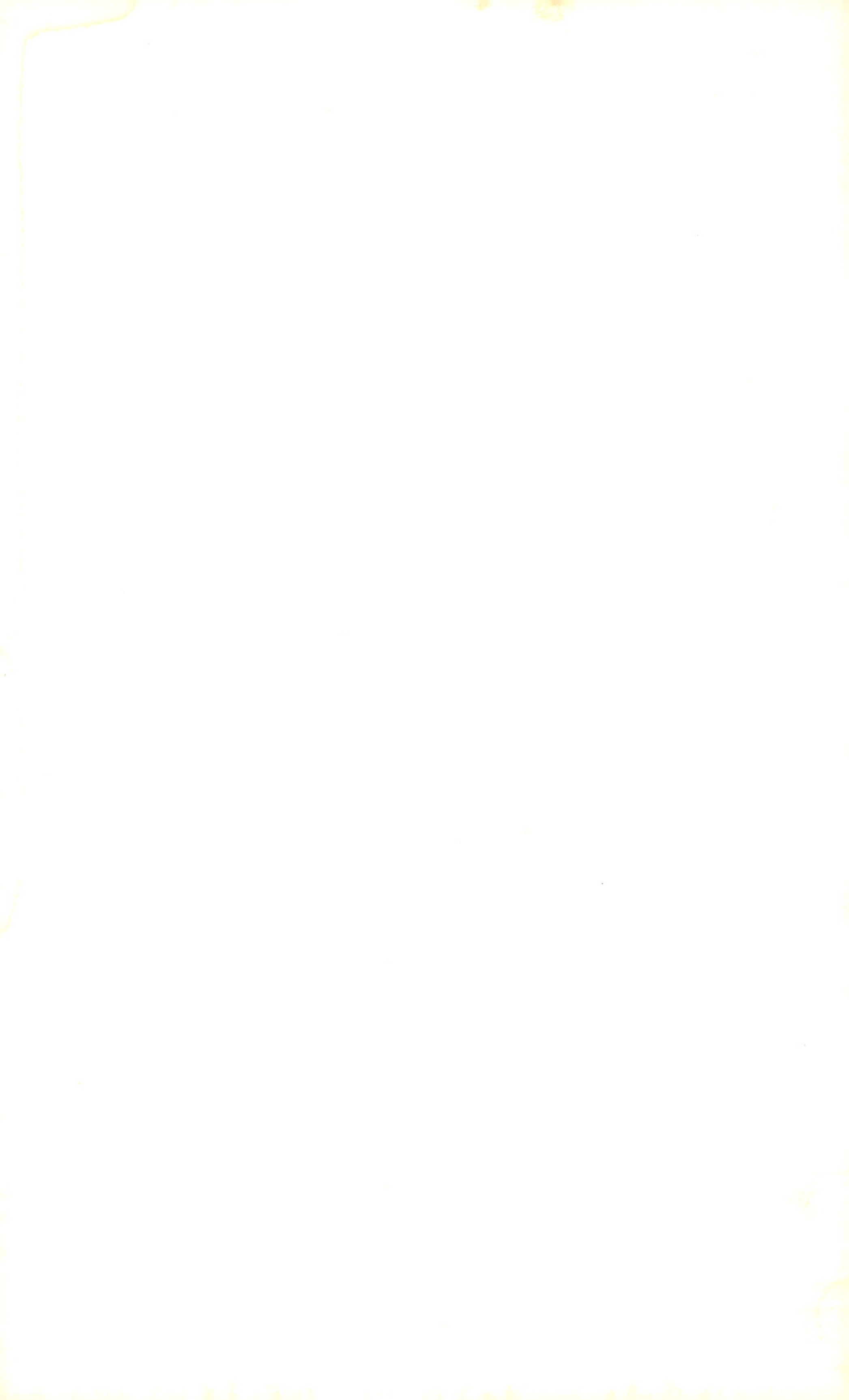

Mainstreams of Medicine

ESSAYS ON THE SOCIAL AND INTELLECTUAL CONTEXT OF MEDICAL PRACTICE

Edited by Lester S. King, M.D.

Introduction by David A. Kronick, Ph.D.

PUBLISHED FOR THE UNIVERSITY OF TEXAS MEDICAL SCHOOL AT SAN ANTONIO BY THE UNIVERSITY OF TEXAS PRESS, AUSTIN & LONDON

International Standard Book Number 0–292–70112–8
Library of Congress Catalog Card Number 78–149564

Type set by G&S Typesetters, Austin
Printed by Capital Printing Company, Austin
Bound by Universal Bookbindery, Inc., San Antonio

FOREWORD

The events and experiences associated with the establishment of a new medical school cannot be catalogued or classified with ease, nor can the whole process be reduced to a mechanical program which can then be used by others to achieve the same results. As is true of many of man's efforts, all of the factors which must be united to produce a new medical school are a product of the region, time, and society which demand this effort. As The University of Texas Medical School at San Antonio was developed, it was evident to several of the faculty (at a time when the total number of faculty was less than twenty) that the traditions of scholarship and dedication to the history and art of medicine, which are a part of the mortar of long established schools, would be too long in development at a new school. In the search for a proper approach, Dr. David A. Kronick, professor of Medical Bibliography, in consultation with Dr. Lester S. King, developed the concept of *Mainstreams of Medicine*. This was not an effort to achieve "instant culture," but rather a means of announcing the birth of a new institution of higher learning to a community that had long awaited such news.

The John and Mary R. Markle Foundation with its chartered objective "to promote the advancement and diffusion of knowledge . . . and . . . the general good of mankind" responded generously to the request for funds to support the series. This medical school is deeply grateful to the Markle Foundation for this support and also for the fact that two of its faculty have the distinction of having earlier been named Scholars in Academic Medicine by the Markle Foundation.

The cooperation of many is acknowledged with appreciation: Dr. Kronick, whose idea it was, and Dr. King, who helped to implement the idea; the staff of KLRN for their assistance in preparing the videotapes; the staff of our own Department of Medical Communications for their participation; Mr. Richard Miller and the Department of Media and Community Information for their assistance with publicity and interviews; the faculty members who served as hosts for our distinguished visitors; and all our students, faculty, staff and fellow citizens who took part in the programs on Sunday afternoons.

Please read this volume with the same pleasure and pride that went into its preparation. You have in your hands a new medical school with its roots in the past and its branches reaching to the future. This is its first product, and I respectfully invite you to share our achievement.

Fitzhugh Carter Pannill, M.D.
Dean, The University of Texas Medical School at San Antonio

EDITOR'S NOTE

Time was when the physician had a quite limited role. He saw sick persons, made diagnoses, and gave proper treatments. To prepare himself for this role he studied certain subjects that eventually came to be known as "basic sciences," and he learned how these related to disease. He learned a fair amount about diseases and how to diagnose them, about patients and how to treat them. But the causes and treatment of disease, which seemed so simple two centuries ago, are no longer simple. With advancing knowledge, the roots of illness are found to be many and far-reaching, penetrating into the physical and mental environment and the social fabric. The physician who wants to understand and treat disease finds himself drawn more and more into peripheral fields. Medical practice, to be effective, must involve all society and not merely the patient.

As medicine becomes more and more complex, the role of the physician changes. As always, he must take care of sick people. But whether he wills it or not, he must also concern himself with problems that even a century ago seemed quite remote, problems of economics and education, of sociology and ethics, of critical judgment, of illusion and reality.

All these aspects are intensely relevant to the physician of the future. How is he to learn about them? At the present time medical schools offer little or no formal education in such subjects, make no premedical requirements. At present the teachers of medicine can only use less formal ways to influence students—encourage them to hear lectures, to pursue appropriate readings. As the mainstream of medicine changes, the student must be encouraged to move with it.

Behind the present volume was the conception of giving medical students—and mature physicians—a wider perspective. The many contributors represent different interests and different points of view. In their professional work, they have all helped to enlarge this perspective and they now share with the reader some of their insights. The separate essays are not intended as a unified text but only as a stimulus—or perhaps I should say an invitation—to appreciate new currents in medicine and to participate therein.

Lester S. King, M.D.

CONTENTS

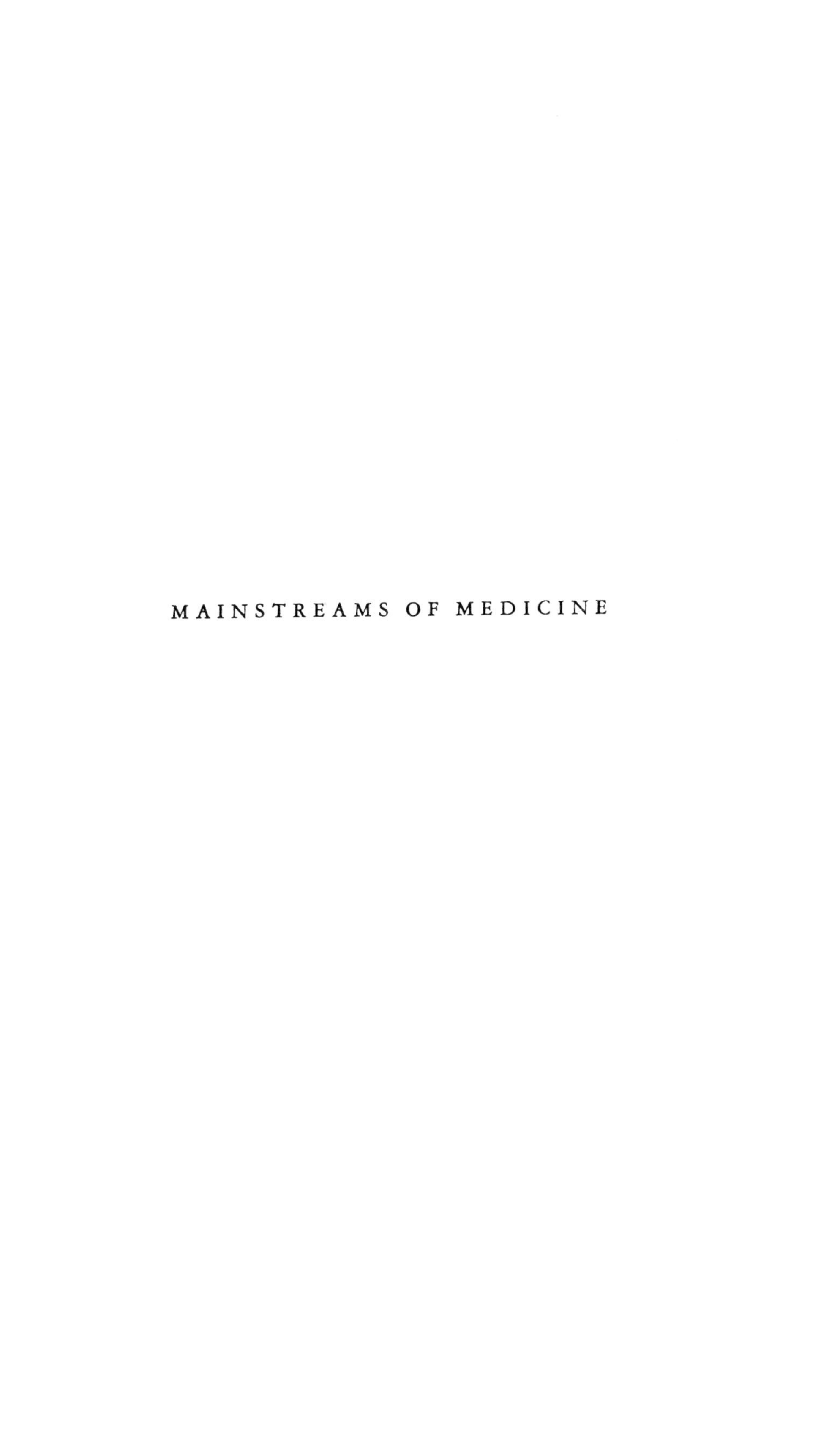

MAINSTREAMS OF MEDICINE

Introduction
Medical Education in Mainstream

DAVID A. KRONICK, Ph.D.

The University of Texas Medical School at San Antonio

THE FACULTY OF A NEW MEDICAL SCHOOL in designing what it hopes will be an innovative curriculum faces a large number of interesting challenges, opportunities, and dilemmas, although the dilemmas very often seem to outweigh either the challenges or the opportunities. The faculty bears a great responsibility, for it will have to put its imprimatur on a student's work and state that this young man or young woman is competent to cope with the ills, the dis-eases, of fellow human beings. A faculty also faces a number of equally urgent but conflicting demands: (1) incorporating into the curriculum as much as possible of the constantly increasing corpus of medical knowledge; (2) recognizing the increasing need for humanizing medical practice, that is, constantly reminding oneself that although medical practice should be informed by science it should be directed by human values, and (3) meeting the constantly increasing demand and need for more physicians.

Some of these dilemmas emerge from the processes of medical teaching and learning and the characteristics of medicine as a science and as an art; but some also derive from the changing conditions of life, the new self-assertiveness of the young, their insistence upon meaningful answers, and resistance to authoritarianism. Today, when medicine is developing increasingly impressive scientific underpinnings, it is becoming more subject to the social processes of stress and change which mark any viable social institution. The medical student today has greater reason for trying to understand these phenomena than students who preceded him, because his new profession is having its social motivations and orientations more critically examined. Physicians are not any more responsible than the rest of us for the general state of amorality so common in our modern society, but physicians are a great deal more socially conspicuous than, say, bankers, lawyers, or accountants. Of all human activities, not many touch man as intimately as that of the physician, nor do many depend so much upon one human being's sensitivity to another human being.

Humanistic Studies

Humanistic studies might seem to be a very important concern of the medical student. On the other hand, medical students frequently give the impression that they have left their humanistic studies behind them as a kind of toy of their childhood. Now that they can literally put their hands into the blood and guts of life they can deal with the very mechanism of man rather than with the pallid representations they knew in their youth. This is a gross exaggeration, of course, since they know very well, if they think about it, that, in order to deal successfully with man (the patient) as a biological entity, they must also deal with him as a sentient and social being.

In the section of the *Etymologies* of Isadore of Seville on medical education, medicine is not classed with the liberal arts because: "The liberal arts comprise single subjects whereas medicine involves all."[1] The medical student can learn as much, sometimes, from a poet as he can from a physiologist about how a man functions as a man. There is a poem by A. E. Housman, for instance, which describes an interesting psychiatric phenomenon:[2]

[1] Loren C. MacKinney, *Early Medieval Medicine* (Baltimore: The Johns Hopkins Press, 1957), p. 96.

[2] Permission to include these lines by A. E. Housman has been granted by The Society of Authors, as the literary representative of the Estate of A. E. Housman, and Jonathan Cape, Ltd., publishers of A. E. Housman's *Col-*

Good creatures, do you love your lives
   And have you ears for sense?
Here is a knife like other knives,
   That cost me eighteen pence.

I need but stick it in my heart
   And down will come the sky,
And earth's foundations will depart
   And all you folk will die.

Where can you find a better evocation of suicide as an act of vindication against a hostile world? Freud expresses this very well when he says: "Imaginative writers are valuable colleagues. In the knowledge of the human heart they are far ahead of us common folk, because they draw on sources that we have not yet made accessible to science."[3] Walt Whitman expresses the idea that to achieve full self-realization man must not only regard himself as a part of nature, but must also learn to live with himself, that to achieve the brotherhood of man, man must first come to terms with himself:[4]

One's-self I sing, a simple separate person
Yet utter the word Democratic, the word En-Masse.

The medical student can even learn something about physician-patient relations from the imaginative literature. Alexander Solzhenitsyn, describing the chief surgeon of the cancer ward making ward rounds, indicates the sensitivity the physician can show toward his patient.[5] At one bedside he is given an X ray which shows an ominous tumorous formation in the iliac region. He holds the film up to the light and nods encouragingly: "That's a very good photo! Very good!"

I have a strong conviction that this kind of sensitivity is also

lected Poems. Copyright 1936 by Barclays Bank Ltd. Copyright © 1964 by Robert E. Symons. Reprinted by permission of Holt, Rinehart and Winston Inc.

3 Alan A. Stone and Sue Smart Stone, eds., *The Abnormal Personality through Literature* (Englewood Cliffs, N.J.: Prentice-Hall, 1966), p. vii.

4 Walt Whitman, "One's-self I Sing," in *Leaves of Grass.*

5 Alexander Solzhenitsyn, *Cancer Ward* (New York: Farrar, Straus and Giroux, 1969).

enhanced by music and art as well as by poetry, literature, and drama. In the face of the growing amount of information in molecular biology, it is impossible, however, to muster up enough courage to argue for these studies as a part of the formal medical curriculum. The students must be reminded that the arts, literature, and music can contribute to their competence as practitioners and they should try not to cut off any avenues of growth in these areas. They have, however, a greater obligation to explore the humanistic studies of philosophy, sociology, and history as they relate to medicine, because these have direct and even urgent relevance to their role as physicians in the community.

Societal Aspects

It is not easy to determine how much of the current unrest in medical education is a part of the general intellectual and social stirrings of our whole society and how much of it grows out of the inherent characteristics of medicine itself. Since medicine is very much involved in society, it is naturally affected by the changes which take place in society. Medicine consists of both science and art, but it is also a social institution, subject to the stresses in our economic and political life. Like our other social institutions it has developed a structure and a system which are not always clearly understood. It is extremely important, therefore, that physicians be aware of the sociology of their profession, especially if they are to make constructive choices about the way medicine evolves, and if the leadership in making these choices will arise from within the profession rather than be imposed upon it.

A strong reciprocal relationship exists between medicine and the society of which it is a part. It is difficult for any element of a culture not to be caught up in the tempo of the times. In my innocence I once made what I thought was an original observation to a musicologist friend of mine. "There must be," I said, "a profound relationship between the work rhythms of a period and the kind of music it produces." We are hardly ever aware of them, because we are part of the tempos ourselves. My friend dismissed my observation by citing a three-volume work in German on the subject, which methodically validates this theory. In the same way our social and economic conditions must influence our ethical judgments and must also profoundly influence our attitudes toward illness, and perhaps even our modes of therapy. We see a terrifying example of this phenomenon in German medicine under Hitler. Alexander has shown how even a small breach in medical ethics led step by step, from the first "rational" decision to deal "pragmatically" with patients having incurable diseases to the death ovens at Dachau.[6] History has some profound lessons to teach us on the ways social, economic, and cultural forces have affected our methods of practicing medicine and of delivering health care.

Obsolescence of Knowledge

The study of history has another great contribution to make to the education of the medical student. Information, we are told, is accruing at a rate faster than we can assimilate it. But what does the process of assimilation involve? Does it mean the development of broad generalizations into which large numbers of discrete observations can be tucked away? Or does it mean the ability to convert our new-won information to practical use? These questions are highly significant for understanding the changes in the scientific bases of medicine which, we are told, are proceeding at an increasing rate. We hear, for instance, that a generation ago a man out of medical school twenty years was still not technically obsolete, but today he may be so after six or seven years.[7] In a sense, someone has observed, medical students in most of their courses are being taught history in the minutest detail.

And here we have other dilemmas of medical teaching: reconciling acceptance with skepticism, or reconciling passing examinations today with learning how to maintain continuity with the developing state of the art, in order to solve medical problems in the future when the student's skills will be put to the test. Medicine

6 Leo Alexander, "Medical Science under Dictatorship," *New Eng. J. Med.* 241 (1949): 39–47.

7 Richard M. Magraw, *Ferment in Medicine* (Philadelphia: W. B. Saunders Co., 1966), p. 3.

began to become scientific when practitioners began to be skeptical of the prevailing medical ideas handed down for generations in their textbooks. The study of the history of medicine is a relatively new discipline. The corpus of medical knowledge was handed down like the teaching of the sacrament, and physicians learned their Galen as schoolboys learned their catechism. "And just as the texts on which the theologians, canon lawyers and classical scholars commented were treated as sacrosanct, as monuments which were to be scrutinized for their meaning, but never changed, so were the medical texts treated."[8] It was only when medicine began to be skeptical of these authoritarian teachings that medicine made substantial progress as a science. Skepticism can be considered a fundamental scientific and medical virtue and one which should be carefully nurtured in the medical student. But to acquire the necessary information to cope with medical problems and, even more important, to pass examinations, students are required to cultivate an attitude of acceptance.

The need of a balance between skepticism and belief is, of course, only a part of a much wider need, that of accommodating oneself to change. Knowledge of history can be a powerful tool to help us achieve the kinds of balance we need in medical education, a balance between skepticism and belief, between innovation and the evaluated and tested answers. History teaches us how to live more comfortably in an environment of uncertainty. It serves also to provide us with some basis from which to regard our own environment from distance in time, so that we may not be completely bound by the prejudices of our period and of our clan. The more we become conscious of the forces that drive us, the more we can harness them toward the achievement of useful goals.

The past has a great deal to teach us. We occupy a habitat that resembles in some ways the habitat of our most remote ancestors. From the earliest humanoid to the most advanced modern man, we are all participants in the human experience. Our community with the past provides us with our only means of continuity with the

[8] Charles H. Talbot, *Medicine in Medieval England* (New York: American Elsevier, 1968), p. 65.

future. The truth about Heraclitus's river is not only that we can never step into it twice, but that the river we step into carries in it the impedimenta, the detritus, it has picked up in its travels.

Mainstreams in Medicine

These, then, were some of the ideas that concerned the core faculty of a new medical school in The University of Texas. With this idea in mind the faculty formulated a proposal to the John and Mary R. Markle Foundation to fund a series of lectures which would have as its objective an examination of "the history of the social and intellectual context of medical practice." Our proposal included the following statements:

> Modern medical education faces problems from the explosive growth of scientific information, rapid obsolescence of knowledge, and the necessity that physicians specialize in order to apply available information. These problems have generated a growing need for generalization and humanization in medicine. . . . In the new curriculum of The University of Texas Medical School at San Antonio it has been proposed to present this historical orientation to entering medical students as a part of a program during the Freshman Year which has been given the title: *Introduction to the Study of Medicine*. . . . The introductory course has been designed as a series of lectures on some of the main themes in the history of medicine. These lectures will show the student that medicine is dynamic and changing; that it has been influenced both by human limitations and human aspirations, and that it is an integral part of the social structure.

We proposed, therefore, in the inaugural year of this medical school, to invite a number of distinguished lecturers: to discuss with the students subjects in keeping with the philosophy and orientation we presented; to lecture on the same subjects in a more formal way to the medical community as a whole; and to contribute toward a collection of essays, which not only will provide a lasting record of the series of lectures, but also will constitute a source to which future students can be referred. Videotape recordings of the lectures were made, to use with the classes of students that follow and to form a part of the school's videotape library.

Through the publication of this series of essays we have, with the help of a number of distinguished collaborators, achieved the final objective of our proposal. Ten videotapes, in color, some in lecture format and some in interview format, were produced, to capture the substance of each of the ten lectures. These were used successfully to form the basis of discussions with the next first-year class and now make up a permanent part of the videotape library of the Medical Communications Department of this institution. The series would not have been possible without the wise and continued counsel of Dr. Lester S. King, who not only shepherded this collection through the press, but also assisted us greatly in the selection of the writers for this volume. We hope it provides the first link in a chain of efforts to maintain not only our medical school's community with the rich heritage of our medical past, but also a continuity with the evolving medical society of the future.

Great Medical Practitioners: A Historical Survey

CHAUNCEY D. LEAKE, Ph.D., L.H.D., Sc.D., LL.D.

The University of California, San Francisco

IT IS DIFFICULT AND PRESUMPTUOUS FOR ME, a scientist primarily and not a physician at all, to try to discuss the inspiration and stimulus to be derived from great medical practitioners. Perhaps I may be excused because my long years have largely been spent in close association with outstanding medical practitioners and I have felt myself part of their training and practice.

In preparing this chapter I thought at first that I would try to analyze the various factors in the art of practicing medicine, the attitudes and moods which might aid physicians in reaping satisfaction from their work—such matters as generous kindliness of feeling and demeanor, cleanliness and neatness of person, courteous and respectful deportment, keen alertness in diagnosing patient and family milieu, and wise and careful judgment in applying all the available and verifiable biomedical knowledge to getting patients well and keeping them so. This analysis might well be illustrated by reference to many distinguished medical practitioners in many different places and times. It might inspire an enthusiastic determination in new and coming physicians to try to follow the rewarding example set by so many capable medical men over so many centuries and in so many lands—as rewarding in subjective individual satisfaction as in social prestige and funds.

Then I thought that I would rather focus attention on a dozen admittedly great medical practitioners whose lives and work in taking good care of sick people could be used as worthy examples for the standards and ideals of medical practice that would be appealing to us. These would not be great scientists, not necessarily significant contributors to our verifiable knowledge of health and disease, but rather great exemplars of the *art* of medicine, who used discriminating judgment wisely and well in applying the knowledge available to them in a way that would promote the welfare of their patients.

These might properly include the revered "Father of Medicine," Hippocrates of Cos (460–375 B.C.), who set standards of medical practice for the ancient Greek world which are still applicable; the respected Muslim-Jewish Moses Maimonides (1135–1204), who so effectively guided the perplexed of his and following times; the gentle French military surgeon, Ambroise Paré (1510–1590), who so humbly but well performed the rough duties expected of him; Thomas Sydenham (1624–1689), the "English Hippocrates," whose practical common sense endeared him to his patients; that great Dutch clinician, Hermann Boerhaave (1668–1738), world renowned for his humanitarian practice; the book- and people-loving Richard Mead (1673–1754), who carried the "gold-headed cane" with effective dignity in his busy London practice; the ethically minded Thomas Percival (1740–1805), whose guidelines for harmonious medical practice were even more a matter of etiquette than of ethics; the always involved Benjamin Rush (1745–1813), signer of the Declaration of Independence, and busiest and best of the many great early Philadelphia physicians; the brilliant Dublin practitioner William Stokes (1804–1878), who learned so much in the tiny Dublin Infirmary of only six beds; the greatest humanist and clinician of our times, William Osler (1849–1919), whose clinical wisdom is already legendary; the dedicated humanitarian and gentle practitioner, Albert Schweitzer (1875–1964), who brought wise medicine, music, philosophy, and hard work to the African jungle; and that "incurable physician," Walter C. Alvarez (1884–), who still gets his greatest joy in taking care of sick and depressed patients, and in writing about it.

As in any selection, so many have to be left out. What about Sir Thomas Browne (1605–1682), famed for his practice and his *Religio Medici*, or that devoted Georgia physician, Crawford W. Long (1815–1878), whose tender concern for his patients led him to forgo the credit for being the first to use modern anesthetics? What about the recent horde of truly heroic physicians who have so well taken care of their patients in far off China, Japan, India, Africa, and the diverse Indies that mortality has been so reduced that we have a global population problem? From such a plethora who can select by name those who have so excelled that their lives may become an inspiration to the young physicians who will follow them?

Art is long, life short, and judgment often faulty, says the first of the famed Hippocratic aphorisms. To make an appropriate selection of specific great medical practitioners whose lives might inspire young people entering the profession is a difficult task. In this discussion I will compromise: I will try to give a historical overview of the ideals and standards, of the tremendous sweep of medicine, with particular reference to a dozen outstanding practitioners whose names I have listed.

The Early Architects of Medicine

The standards and ideals of modern health professionals derive from antiquity: from Chinese formalism, Hindu etiquette, Sumerian division of labor, and Egyptian practicality. The early Greek Asklepiads were archetypes of gentle physicians. In the Hippocratic writings are clear injunctions for humanistic and humanitarian relations with patients, for high regard for the dignity of the individual, and for decent dealings with all. In the Hippocratic *Oath*, in *The Law*, and other writings, there are many featured phrases which have a pleasant modern sound, perhaps because they are so deeply a part of the long humanistic tradition of the health professions.

Pride in the art of medicine has been part of medical practice from its beginning. Even the ancient Greeks fully realized the danger of pride turning into arrogance, and ever cautioned lest this hubris might not bring its nemesis. This professional pride has been an ever-present inspiration to all the health professions, from nursing (the earliest), to medicine and surgery, to dentistry, to pharmacy, to veterinary medicine, and now to public health and the many health services. Here, as Sir William Osler emphasized for us, our most sophisticated modernism cannot surpass the medical wisdom of antiquity.

While this idealistic spirit may have faltered in the hard realities of Rome, as in our own time, and then in the degradation of the "Dark Ages," it was well developed among Muslim physicians and was warmly welcomed again in medieval Europe. Hospitals were established and were well operated and supported. Nursing, medicine, and pharmacy were practiced for the welfare of patients, with an art that partially compensated for the appalling ignorance of the causes of infectious and metabolic diseases, which so strongly kept down population pressures. The relative cleanliness and solicitous care shown in the hospitals was in marked contrast to the filth and cruelty in the villages and cities.

Moses Maimonides may be taken as the most worthy example of idealistic medical practice of this era. His learning embraced both the grand Jewish tradition and the rich Muslim culture. Born in Spanish Córdoba, where his memory as a great medical practitioner is still revered, he went east to Cairo. His skill was so outstanding that he became physician to the renowned Saladin (1137–1193), whose magnanimity shamed the Crusaders. His treatise on personal hygiene resulted from his experience with the Sultan and, translated into Latin as *Tractatus de Regimine Sanitatis*, it was among the first printed medical books (Florence, 1478). His humanistic zeal was expressed in his well-known *Guide for the Perplexed.* The Prayer of Maimonides remains a clear call to the idealism and conscience of all members of the health professions and services.

During the exciting and vigorous Renaissance, it seems to me that the best example of the idealistic, devoted, and humane medical practitioner was the brilliant French military surgeon, Ambroise Paré. Starting as a barber, he became an orderly at the famed Hôtel-Dieu in Paris, and then went with the armies to care for the wounded. His solid sense, skill, and bravery made him the founder of modern surgery, although he was scorned by the entrenched faculty. He taught and wrote in French, instead of the academic Latin with which he was unfamiliar, and he applied the newly described human anatomy of Andreas Vesalius (1514–1564) to practical surgery. Beloved by his comrades, he told many tales of his care for them, modestly stating that, while he treated them, God cured them. Busy though he was in tough fighting and in the daily care of the injured and dying, Paré always seems to have had the time to be gentle and considerate with his patients. He kept detailed records of his individual patients, referring to them by name, thus remembering that they were, first of all, human beings. These accounts in his *Divers Journeys* still give a vivid picture of the skilled and wise surgeon that he was.

In moving to the rising ferment of intellectual energy in seventeenth-century Europe, one finds a great medical practitioner who returned to Hippocratic wisdom in the effective care of his patients. Thomas Sydenham, says Fielding Garrison, "ennobled the practice of physic through those qualities of piety, good humor, and good sense which Edmund Burke declared to be the genius of the English race." Burke was, of course, also an Englishman, but Sydenham was beyond race or place, as a great man who took superlative care of his sick patients. He had no part in the medical science of his time, but was supreme in its art. He insisted that theories help little at the bedside of a sick person, but that wide experience and sharp observation will be the best guides to clinical success. His idea of the natural course of a disease in a sick person was coupled with the Hippocratic notion of the *vis medicatrix naturae*, and he knew that a hopeful sick person would tend to get well regardless of what a physician might do. In sharing his observational skill with his colleagues through his writings, Sydenham forced recognition of the clear differences between many closely related diseases.

The medical transition from the many scientific discoveries of the seventeenth century to the enlightened practice of the eighteenth century was marked especially by Hermann Boerhaave, the greatest clinical teacher since Hippocrates. Although he made no scientific discoveries himself, he was simply the most outstanding physician of his time, and patients came to his Leiden home from all over the world, even from China and the Americas. While it was as a teacher that he excelled, his skill in teaching was derived from his detailed study of his individual patients. Medical students, too, came in droves, from all over the world, to his brilliant lectures, and thus carried his clinical wisdom everywhere.

Transition to Our Own Times

Much of what is characteristic of medicine in our United States comes from eighteenth-century English practice, quite as Latin American medical practice comes from Madrid and Paris. The care of the sick in eighteenth-century England was professionally organized among physicians, surgeons, and apothecaries, with rather rigid social distinction. The physicians often came from landed families, with inherited incomes. In such aristocratic families it was the custom for the first son to become a clergyman, the second a physician, the third a lawyer, and the fourth a military man. The physician went to Oxford or Cambridge and received an M.D. degree.

The apothecaries were tradesmen, who dispensed drugs, but also treated minor illnesses. They had their own guild and could be licensed after examination, but they had no university degree. Ordinarily, a sick person would first go to an apothecary, who might give some drug therapy after simple questioning or inspection. If the situation was beyond his ability he was usually wise enough to send the sick person to consult the physician, who would assume responsibility and make the important decisions. This system worked fairly well in practice for quite a while.

The surgeons generally came from middle-class or poor families and learned by apprenticeship. Hospital training was available, as was special didactic work in London anatomy schools. Young surgeons had stiff examinations to pass before they would be licensed by the Royal College of Surgeons. The surgeons did not need a university degree, and English surgeons still prefer to be called "mister."

The epitome of the conscientious eighteenth-century English

physician was Richard Mead, famed for his courtly manner, his fine library, and his high sense of *noblesse oblige*. Taught first by Boerhaave in Leiden, Mead received his M.D. degree at Padua. A dissenter from the established church, Mead was nevertheless a deeply religious man and won the respect of all. His patients ranged from the most humble to Queen Anne herself, and he was careful in his attention to the sick who sought his advice at any and all times. How he found time for literary activity is a puzzle, but he did write well. Asked to guide the people against the plague, he wrote *A Short Discourse Concerning Pestilential Contagion* (London, 1720), which laid the background for the later English public health system. Mead was the second carrier of the famed "gold-headed cane," having inherited it from his mentor, John Radcliffe (1650–1714), the popular physician whose fortune made possible the Radcliffe Library, Infirmary, and Observatory at Oxford.

This gold-headed cane became the symbol of devoted English medical practice. It reposes in the Library of the Royal College of Physicians in London, to which it was bequeathed by the widow of the great pathologist Matthew Baillie (1761–1823). In 1827 there appeared a delightful book entitled *The Gold-Headed Cane*, published by John Murray in London. It purported to be the autobiography of the cane. Actually, it was written by William Macmichael (1784–1839), the registrar of the college. It has gone into many editions and portrays the cultural idealism expected of a dedicated medical practitioner.

The well-structured pattern of medical practice in eighteenth-century England was badly battered in the reckless Industrial Revolution which ushered in the machine age. People flocked to the cities; the ancient rural agricultural equilibrium was disrupted; slums appeared as part of the exploitation of workers, and there was appalling misery and sickness. Hospitals and infirmaries had to be provided. There was much jealous friction among physicians, surgeons, and apothecaries as to which group would dominate the scene, control the hospitals, and get credit for caring adequately for the sick. In this unsatisfactory situation there appeared a guidebook for appropriate conduct and decent interpersonal relationships among members of these professional groups, their patients, and the general public. This was the work of an excellent and sensitive medical practitioner, Thomas Percival, of Manchester, where the turmoil and distress of industrialization were especially serious.

Percival, who was a kindly gentleman as well as a keen physician, probably realized that a guideline for decent conduct among the different kinds of members of the health professions was a simple book of etiquette, a standard for interpersonal relations. He was persuaded to call it *Medical Ethics*. This title has since caused much confusion, as the book does not really consider the basic moral questions of medical practice, which we are only now beginning to explore—questions involving abortion, the right of a patient to know the truth or to choose not to live, euthanasia, birth control, and human experimentation.

Percival's *Medical Ethics* had great influence in the frontier conditions in the United States. The population expansion called for many more physicians than the older, well-established schools could supply. New schools sprouted in the frontier cities. The standards of medical education and of practice declined. An idealistic medical teacher at the then far-western Transylvania Medical School, in Lexington, Kentucky, Samuel Brown (1769–1830), thought he could improve matters by founding a medical fraternity for an elite who would uphold high standards of medical practice. The Kappa Lambda Society of Aesculapius was formed about 1819 and soon had chapters in all major American cities. It upheld the standards of decency of Percival's code. Its growing power made it a target for sharp criticism, and it gradually disappeared around 1839.

Unsatisfactory conditions of medical education and practice continued, and in 1846 the situation was serious enough to persuade the outstanding physicians in the country to organize the American Medical Association. Almost its first action was to adopt Percival's *Medical Ethics* as its code of etiquette. This choice made it possible for the conservative physicians to enforce their point of view among their colleagues under pain of expulsion from their respective local medical societies.

The situation became slightly ridiculous in connection with consultation. The "homeopathic" physicians, following the gentle practice but absurd theories of Samuel Christian Hahnemann (1755–1843), were very popular and successful. Actually the therapy was chiefly a placebo, for sick people tend to get well if left alone. The regular physicians were not supposed to consult with homeopathic physicians. This foolish situation even split the New York State Medical Society into competing factions.

In 1903 the rigid "Code" of Ethics was changed to a more reasonable set of "Principles," but was still an etiquette guide, often with conflicting rules. Finally, in 1957, a simple set of ten generalities for decent conduct was adopted. Now we can properly distinguish etiquette from basic moral problems of medical practice and discuss the latter in relation to the various theories of ethics which have been proposed over the centuries.

The ablest, most popular, and most conscientious American physician of the late eighteenth and early nineteenth century was Benjamin Rush, with a humanistic training from Princeton and a medical education partly from an apprenticeship in Philadelphia and partly from the University of Edinburgh, where he received his M.D. degree. He was a signer of the Declaration of Independence and served as a physician in the Revolutionary army. With high social idealism he propagandized against slavery, war, alcoholism, and the death penalty. His was a pioneering interest in mental disorders, and his clinical skill was well recognized. He founded the first public dispensary in our country in 1786, taught brilliantly at the University of Pennsylvania Medical School, and wrote clearly on various diseases. Beloved by his patients, he stayed with them during the terrible yellow fever epidemic of 1793, taking care of over a hundred a day.

It has always thrilled me to think of the great practicing physicians who, during the first part of the nineteenth century, did so well in Dublin in their tiny hospital. There they demonstrated that careful study of each patient is much more rewarding than trying to get broad clinical experience by seeing so many patients in a huge hospital that one becomes easily confused. These Dubliners described what they saw so well that their names are part of every physician's vocabulary: John Cheyne (1777–1836) of Cheyne-Stokes respiration; Robert Adams (1791–1875) of Stokes-Adams syndrome; Abraham Colles (1773–1843) of Colles's fracture; Robert Graves (1796–1853) of Graves' disease; Sir Dominic Corrigan (1802–1880) of Corrigan pulse; and William Wallace (1791–1837), of Wallace's drops. Wallace introduced the saturated solution of potassium iodide by mouth for tertiary syphilis with such success as to suggest the German dictum, "Wenn man weisst nicht wo, weder, oder warum, dann gibt man Kal Iodium."

The great practicing physician of this group, however, was William Stokes, who so well carried on his father's skill. Stokes developed the stethoscope, first used by the great French physician René Laennec (1781–1826). Stokes was renowned for his solicitous care of poor patients. In the Dublin epidemic of typhus fever in 1826, he contracted the disease himself, but continued his ministrations to those others already afflicted. Like his colleagues, he was famed for his knowledge and skill in treatment of cardiac disorders, and his name is associated with heart block. Stokes made his pupils handle patients themselves and stopped the then common abuse and neglect of hospitalized sick.

Modern Times

Among the greatest physicians of our time was Sir William Osler. Anyone reading his monumental biography, written by Harvey Cushing (1869–1939), himself one of the greatest surgeons of our day, would certainly agree. Osler was professor of Medicine successively at McGill University, the University of Pennsylvania, The Johns Hopkins University, and Oxford University. A scintillating bedside teacher, he was a most beloved practicing physician, busy from early morning to late at night with his patients, his students, and his superb humanistic writing. His textbook of medicine has become a classic. His contributions to the history of medicine are great, and he delighted in writing vivid accounts of great physicians, as well as of humble and devoted practitioners, such as "An Alabama Student." His memorable special lectures remain inspiring, and his magnificent library of great medical classics is one of the treasures of McGill, superbly housed and elaborately catalogued. Renowned as a practicing physician, a wise historian, a fun-loving man, a great humanist, and a skilled bibliographer, Osler is the epitome of an ideal practicing physician.

Famous the world over for his devotion to his African jungle patients is Albert Schweitzer, "prophet in the wilderness," as he is called by his biographer, Hermann Hagedorn. First a theologian highly regarded in his native Alsace and in all Europe and also a brilliant musician and organist, Schweitzer decided to study medicine and to devote his life to the care of the sick in jungle Africa. With his wife's help, he accomplished this goal, establishing the famed hospital in Lambaréné. This hospital, built by his patients under his direction, was miserable by our standards, but great in its ministration to the sick natives of a huge area. Active from dawn to midnight, Schweitzer set an example of patient care. Making his patients and their families work to keep the hospital running, Schweitzer won their respect and affection. Meanwhile, he continued his theological and musical activities and obtained worldwide support for his medical endeavors. Although he made no contributions to medical knowledge, he did extend modern medical care to an underdeveloped people. He adjusted the operation of his hospital to the conditions in which he had to work, and he reaped enormous satisfaction from his success. His was medical practice that was simple, effective, at its best.

Now we are in the present. Whom should I select among living physicians to round out a dozen great practicing physicians of all historic time? Such a choice is precarious for many reasons. Yet, of all the practicing physicians I have known—and they are many, in this country and abroad—the one who has come closest, in my opinion, to lifelong devotion to the welfare of his patients, to an idealistic appreciation of a practicing physician's responsibility, and to a humanistic regard for public understanding of what medicine is about must be that "incurable physician," as he has described himself, Walter C. Alvarez, of Chicago.

Walter Alvarez was born in 1884, the son of a remarkable physician from whom he received a wealth of wisdom as a youth in the calm loveliness of Hawaii. He was trained well, and as an intern went through the excitement of the disastrous 1906 earthquake and fire in San Francisco. In his career he went from saddlebag practice in Mexico to productive laboratory studies on gastroenterology at the University of California and at Harvard, and then to the Mayo Clinic. There he developed his reputation as a careful and kindly physician. His wisdom has been distilled in many important volumes, notably on gastroenterology, neuroses, and "little strokes." Always eager to share his experience, he undertook editorial writing for medical periodicals and then pioneered a medical column issued daily in newspapers all over the world. An idealistic, outgoing person, he has given his opinion frankly and honestly. His wisdom has helped greatly in our modern understanding of sexual problems in relation to medicine. At a time when most physicians would have long since retired, he has kept amazingly young in active practice. His life is a model for physicians in our turbulent modern times.

Each of the men I have mentioned exemplifies the best attributes of a worthy practicing physician. In each of them there was a rich store of scientific knowledge and of experience with people in sickness and in health. From this knowledge and experience a keen artistic judgment could select that which could be applied effectively to the welfare of the individual patient. In each of these physicians the science and art of medicine were wedded. In each of them was a love of his work, which, as the Hippocratic writer indicated, is always associated with a love of humanity. In each of them was ever present humility before the unknown, zeal for understanding, tenderness in spirit, devotion to responsibility, and joy in living. In their lives may be found inspiration to solid endeavor for medical students and practicing physicians. In each can be found an enthusiasm which, if caught early as an infection, might immunize medical students and practicing physicians evermore against despair, depression, or disillusionment. For each of these practicing physicians it is his enthusiasm which has made life so well worth living.

SOME REFERENCES FOR PLEASURABLE READING

GENERAL:

F. H. Garrison. *History of Medicine.* 4th edition, reprinted. Philadelphia: W. B. Saunders Co., 1929.

Lester S. King. *The Medical World of the Eighteenth Century.* Chicago: University of Chicago Press, 1958.

HIPPOCRATES:

The Genuine Works of Hippocrates. Trans. Francis Adams. London, 1849 (frequently reprinted, as, New York: Dover Publications, 2 vols., n.d.).

The Medical Works of Hippocrates. Trans. J. Chadwick and W. N. Mann. Springfield, Ill.: Charles C Thomas, Publisher, 1950.

MAIMONIDES:

The Preservation of Youth. Trans. H. L. Gordon. New York: Philosophical Library, 1958.

Two Treatises on the Regimen of Health. Trans. A. Bar-Sela, Hebbell Hoff, and E. Faris. Philadelphia: American Philosophical Society, 1964.

Treatise on Poisons and Their Antidotes. Trans. Suessman Munter. Philadelphia: J. B. Lippincott Co., 1966.

PARÉ:

The Apologie & Treatise of Ambroise Paré. Ed. G. Keynes. Chicago: University of Chicago Press, 1952 (reprinted, N.Y.: Dover Publications, 1968).

Wallace B. Hamby. *Ambroise Paré, Surgeon of the Renaissance.* St. Louis: Warren H. Green, 1967.

SYDENHAM:

The Works of Thomas Sydenham. Trans. R. G. Latham. 2 vols., London: The Sydenham Society, 1848.

K. Dewhurst. *Dr. Thomas Sydenham 1624–1689.* Berkeley: University of California Press, 1966.

BOERHAAVE:

G. A. Lindeboom. *Hermann Boerhaave: The Man and His Work*. London: Methuen, 1968.

MEAD:

W. Macmichael. *The Gold-Headed Cane*. 7th edition. Springfield, Ill.: Charles C Thomas, 1953.

PERCIVAL:

Percival's Medical Ethics. Ed. C. D. Leake. Baltimore: Williams & Wilkins, 1927.

RUSH:

The Autobiography of Benjamin Rush. Ed. G. W. Corner. Princeton: Princeton University Press, 1948.

Benjamin Rush, Medical Inquiries and Observations. Reprint. New York: Hafner, 1962.

STOKES:

William Stokes. *William Stokes: His Life and Work*. London: T. Unwin, 1898.

OSLER:

Aequiminitas and Other Essays. Ed. Paul D. White. New York: Norton, 1963.

An Alabama Student and Other Biographical Essays. New York: Oxford University Press, 1929.

The Old Humanities and the New Science. London: John Murray, 1919.

Aphorisms from Osler's Bedside Teaching. Ed. W. B. Bean. New York: H. Schuman, 1950.

Harvey Cushing. *The Life of Sir William Osler*. 2 vols. New York: Oxford University Press, 1925 (available in single-volume reprint).

"William Osler: Commemorative Issue," *JAMA* 210 (Dec. 22, 1969): 2213–2269 (16 contributions by various authors).

SCHWEITZER:

On the Edge of the Primeval Forest. New York: Macmillan Co., 1948.

Out of My Life and Thought. New York: Henry Holt, 1949.

H. Hagedorn. *Albert Schweitzer, Prophet in the Wilderness*. New York: Collier Paperback, 1962.

ALVAREZ:

Incurable Physician: An Autobiography. Englewood Cliffs, N.J.: Prentice-Hall, 1963.

Little Strokes. Philadelphia: J. B. Lippincott Co., 1966.

NOTE: Most of these items were displayed, with descriptive notes, by David Kronick, the Librarian at The University of Texas Medical School at San Antonio, when I gave my address. I am grateful for his interest and enthusiasm.

C.D.L.

Medicine as a Function of Society

GEORGE ROSEN, M.D.
Department of the History of Medicine
Yale University

I

MAN IS A SOCIAL BEING. It is a characteristic of human beings to associate with each other for mutual protection and advantage. Throughout history, men living in larger or smaller groups have had to take account in various ways of health problems that arise from the biological attributes and needs of their fellows.

As long as man has lived on earth, sickness has plagued him. Disease is associated with life, and man everywhere endeavors to deal with it as best he can. Studies in paleopathology have shown not only the antiquity of disease, but also its occurrence in the same basic biologic forms, such as infection and infestation, disturbances of development and metabolism, traumatism and neoplasia.[1] For example, schistosomiasis, prevalent in Egypt today, has been found in the kidneys of Egyptians who lived 3,000 years ago, and tuberculosis

[1] Adolph H. Schultz, "Notes on Diseases and Healed Fractures of Wild Apes and Their Bearing on the Antiquity of Pathological Conditions in Man," *Bull. Hist. Med.* 7 (1939): 571–582; D. Brothwell, "The Palaeopathology of Early British Man," *J. Royal Anthropol. Inst.* 91 (1961): 318–344; S. Jarcho, "Lead in the Bones of Prehistoric Lead-Glaze Potters," *Amer. Antiq.* 30 (1964): 94–96.

of the spine has been diagnosed in the skeletal remains of pre-Columbian Indians.[2]

But while these basic types have not changed, the incidence and prevalence of illnesses involving such processes have varied from time to time and place to place. Our illnesses and accidents reflect the world in which we live, what we do in it and with it. Caisson disease and welder's conjunctivitis occur as a result of occupational activity, of certain ways of earning a living. Bunions and nylon dermatitis, or dermatitis due to makeup, are related to fashions in dress and cosmetics. Tennis elbow is a recreational hazard in a society where tennis is played. Scurvy and rickets tell us a good deal about diet, living conditions, social class, and the like. This is true of both the present and the past. The occurrence of disease in a given population at a particular time exhibits a characteristic pattern defined by causation, morbidity, and mortality, as related to age, sex, social class, occupation, mode of life, and, more generally, to the culture and psychology of a society. The pattern of disease which occurs in any group of people is not a matter of chance. Broadly speaking, it is associated with the level of social and technical development of the population and is significantly related to the values prevailing in the group. It is an expression of interaction with the environment in its various facets. Insofar, then, as disease arises from, or affects, the social conditions or relations under which men live, it is a social phenomenon and is completely comprehensible only within a biosocial context. In these terms, the history of disease is to be seen as more than the study of discrete clinical entities; it becomes the delineation of the disease patterns characteristic of certain historical periods and societies and of the factors and processes that led to their change in time and space.

This approach may be illustrated by several examples. Recently, Odin Anderson and I applied the concept of disease patterns in an analysis of the idea of preventive medicine. We felt that in the history of Europe over the past 1,000 years there were five periods, in

[2] M. A. Ruffer, *Studies in the Palaeopathology of Egypt* (Chicago: University of Chicago Press, 1921), pp. 17–19.

each of which one or two diseases were most characteristic. Of these, for example, we felt that the period from the end of the fifteenth century into the first half of the nineteenth century was dominated by louse-borne diseases and syphilis, but that these were replaced in the nineteenth century as major health problems by typhoid fever and cholera. Finally, we pointed out that the leading health problems of fifty years ago have been replaced by cancer, heart disease, and accidents. In fact, we concluded that "if the leading causes of death in an area *are* heart disease and cancer, one can be assured that the area has kept abreast of modern medicine and its application."[3]

The disease pattern of a period, of a community, or of an area may be significant also because of its relation to historical and social change. In 1849 the pathologist Rudolf Virchow elaborated a theory of epidemic disease as a manifestation of social and cultural maladjustment. He pointed out that with the dawning of new historical periods "epidemic diseases exhibiting a hitherto unknown character appear and disappear, often without leaving a trace. As cases in point take leprosy and the English sweat."[4] Virchow chose two apposite diseases to illustrate his theory, but he might have picked others, for with the opening of the modern period the disease picture of Europe changed significantly. Diseases hitherto widely prevalent, such as leprosy, diminished in importance and made way for new or at least previously unnoticed pestilential scourges. Among the diseases that were observed for the first time or were studied in a more precise way during the sixteenth and seventeenth centuries were the English sweat, typhus fever, scurvy, some of the acute exanthemata, such as scarlet fever and chicken pox, and the disease

[3] Odin W. Anderson and George Rosen, *An Examination of the Concept of Preventive Medicine*, Health Information Research Series, no. 12 (New York, 1960), pp. 18–19.

[4] Rudolf Virchow, *Die Einheitsbestrebungen in der wissenschaftlichen Medicin* (Berlin: G. Reimer, 1849), pp. 47–48; *idem*, "Die Epidemien von 1848, Gelesen in der Jahressitzung der Gesellschaft für wissenschaftliche Medicin am 27. November, 1848," *Archiv für pathologische Anatomie und Physiologie und für klinische Medicin* 3 (1851): 3–12.

that was to become a major health problem from the Renaissance to our time—syphilis.

Scurvy, the black death of the sea, is illustrative of this theme. The stories of the geographic discoveries of the fifteenth and sixteenth centuries are familiar. However, the world grown more spacious yielded fresh and unanticipated problems. The sea routes to the Far East and the New World involved longer voyages than had ever been undertaken before, and these directed attention to new health problems. On the long voyages the greatest enemy of the sailor was scurvy, due essentially to a diet deficient in or devoid of vitamin C. Scurvy was not a new disease. It had been observed during the Middle Ages in besieged towns when the supply of fresh provisions was cut off, or in times of scarcity. The disease became an acute problem, however, just as soon as the seafarers of western Europe ventured out into the Atlantic. The Portuguese were among the first to face the ravages of scurvy. English experience with this scourge of seamen began about the middle of the sixteenth century on early voyages to Africa. For more than two hundred years scurvy continued to be a widespread disease among seamen. Lord Anson's voyage around the world (1740–1744) was one of the more disastrous experiences during this period. One year after sailing from England, 65 per cent of the crews of Anson's three ships had perished, chiefly from scurvy.[5]

As this discussion implies, the pattern or distribution of disease in a period or an area is significant on several grounds. Not only is it related to historical developments, but it is also intimately linked to the social situation of those affected by disease. Pellagra is a case in point. How pellagra could be prevented or cured was known by 1920, yet in 1934 the disease caused 3,602 deaths in the United States, with about 20 reported cases for each death. The reason lay not so much in a lack of knowledge, but rather in the economic factors that affected the dietary of the cotton-raising South. Joseph

[5] George Anson, *A Voyage Round the World* (1748), comp. Richard Walter, rev. edn., Everymans Library (London: J. M. Dent, 1911), pp. xv–xvii.

Goldberger, who elucidated the etiology of pellagra, studied the role of economic and social factors in its causation.[6] With Edgar Sydenstricker he carried out a series of classic studies in the social epidemiology of pellagra in cotton-mill villages and among tenant farmers. An unmistakable inverse correlation between family income and pellagra incidence was demonstrated. As income increased, the pellagra rate declined. However, income was not the only factor involved. Food supply and dietary habits played important roles as well. Given the restricted food pattern of the poorer class in the South, when families in mill villages were restricted to the mill store or commissary during the late winter or spring because of the absence of other sources of supply, pellagra was almost inevitable. Goldberger could recommend keeping cows and chickens, and planting gardens, but he could not change the economics of the situation. As he wrote in 1927, referring to the rural population: "It is necessary to keep in mind two considerations of essential importance. The first is that the economic status of this population is bound up in the tenant system, which, in turn, is involved in single-crop agricultural production and the speculative character of agricultural finance as it is practiced in this area, the seasonal fluctuation in income of the tenant . . . and other factors of an economic nature."[7]

Not only is disease related causally to the social situation of a given population and its members, but also the health care received is a reflection of the structure of society, and particularly of its class divisions. Thus, Plato in the *Republic* has Socrates say to Glaucon, "When a carpenter is ill he asks the physician for a rough-and-ready cure. An emetic, a purge, a cautery, or the knife—that is the remedy for him. But if someone prescribes for him a course of dietetics or tells him to wrap his head up and keep himself warm, he replies at once that he has no time to be ill, that he sees no good in a life that is spent in nursing his disease to the neglect of his customary employment. He therefore bids the doctor good-bye, resumes his

[6] *Goldberger on Pellagra*, ed. Milton Terris (Baton Rouge: Louisiana State University Press, 1964), pp. 113–291.

[7] *Ibid.*, p. 290.

ordinary way of life, and either gets well, lives, and does his business or, if his constitution fails, he dies and is rid of his troubles."[8]

A pertinent comment on the same point was made by Bernardino Ramazzini in 1713. Concerning medical care for brickmakers he remarked, "Workers of this sort are mostly of the peasant class; so, when they are attacked by fever they betake themselves to their huts and leave the affair entirely to nature; or else they are carried off to hospitals and there are treated, like everybody else, with the usual remedies, purging and venesection. For the doctors know nothing of the mode of life of these workers, who are exhausted and prostrated by increasing toil." Furthermore, he adds, "for these wretched workers the best remedy would be a fresh-water bath at the earliest stage when they begin to have fever; for their bodies are rough and dry with dirt, and by moistening the skin and opening the pores, the fever would be given an outlet."[9]

That the differential provision of medical care by social class is still a fact of life can easily be confirmed. Just over a decade ago Hollingshead and Redlich, in their study *Social Class and Mental Illness*, produced evidence to show that social class is related significantly to the prevalence of treated psychiatric disorders, the types of treated psychiatric disorders, and the kind of therapy administered. A very recent study by Duff and Hollingshead, entitled *Sickness and Society*, only adds more evidence to support the general proposition that medical care is not provided strictly in terms of need, and that it is governed to a considerable degree by other factors.

The same point applies as well to age categories. For example, before the nineteenth century, when a high infant mortality prevailed, the attitude toward childhood was different from that generally accepted today in technically advanced societies.[10] "I lost two

[8] Plato *Republic* 406D.

[9] Bernardino Ramazzini, *Diseases of Workers*, the Latin Text of 1713, revised with translation and notes by Wilmer Cave Wright (Chicago: University of Chicago Press, 1940), p. 449.

[10] Lynn Thorndike, "Fifteenth Century Patients," *Bull. Hist. Med.* 28 (1954): 252–258; Dean Lockwood, *Ugo Benzi: Medieval Philosopher and Physician 1376–1439* (Chicago: University of Chicago Press, 1951), pp. 67–

or three children as nurslings," wrote Montaigne, "not without regret but without great grief." Children hardly counted until they had reached an age of probable survival. Certain *consilia* of physicians at the end of the medieval period seem to reflect this attitude and situation. Thus, among 309 *consilia* of Bartolomeo de Montagnana (d. 1460), 19 concern adolescents, 5 boys, 2 young children, and only one an infant. Similarly, among over 100 *consilia* of Ugo Benzi (1376–1439), one concerns a boy of ten, another a child of two and a half. Obviously, such evidence is only suggestive, but it does point to the relevance of social structure and values in the provision of health care.

To put the problem more generally, whether a given society emphasizes a given stage of biological maturation depends on historical and cultural factors. In medieval Europe, infancy ended at about the age of six or seven, and the individual was then considered an adult. The concept of childhood emerged gradually during the seventeenth and eighteenth centuries. Even more recent in origin is the concept of adolescence, which dates from the nineteenth and twentieth centuries. In other words, the stages of the life cycle depend not only on physiological maturation, but even more on the way in which a society structures social roles by age. Such changing concepts are reflected in other social institutions, and have an impact on them, for example, in the organization and provision of medical care. Instances in point are the medical specialties of pediatrics and geriatrics, and the various institutional arrangements connected with them.

II

The social group not only defines who receives medical care and in what form, but it also establishes special institutions for the sick. Illness creates dependency. The sick need not only medical treatment, but also personal care and shelter. Throughout history, societies have accepted such needs as a responsibility of group life and

68, 264–266, 309; Philippe Ariès, *L'Enfant et la vie familiale sous l'ancien régime* (Paris: Plon, 1960), p. 29.

have created various institutions to provide the services deemed necessary. One of these institutions, the hospital, is today a cornerstone of any modern system of health care. Arrangements to provide for the needs of the sick have always been intimately linked with the varying political, economic, social, and cultural conditions that govern the life of man in society. Whether man lived in a city or on the land, whether he suffered scarcity or enjoyed abundance, how he saw his fellow men and how they looked upon him, the religion he practiced and the values he prized, the learning, sciences, and arts that gave shape to his society—all have affected the development of the hospital, the form it has achieved, the services it has provided, and the impact it has had on the community and on specific groups in it. In terms of these facets, the hospital has to be seen as an organ of society, sharing certain of its basic characteristics, changing as the society of which it is a part is transformed, and, in turn, exerting an influence on social groups and situations.

At various periods in history the need to care for the sick and the disabled, the needy and the dependent, has crystallized sufficiently in terms of attitude and practice so that one can speak of institutional models characteristic of certain periods and societies. In this sense the history of the hospital may be seen in terms of certain types that have predominated in given historical periods. Although knowledge concerning the healing shrines and the secular healing institutions of antiquity is too incomplete for any generalizations, this is not the case for the medieval period.

The medieval hospital in its varied forms was essentially an ecclesiastical institution. While the provision of medical care was one of its functions, it was created primarily on religious and spiritual values as a philanthropic institution, an agency of poor relief. Generally speaking, the hospital was a religious house in which the nursing personnel united as a vocational community under a religious rule.[11] A medical staff and its activities are central to the

[11] Leon le Grand, *Statuts d'hôtels-Dieu et de léproseries: Recueil de textes du* XIIe *au* XIVe *siècles* (Paris: Alphonse Picard et Fils, 1901); Dorothy-Louise Mackay, *Les Hôpitaux et la charité à Paris au* XIIIe *siècle* (Paris: Honoré Champion, 1923), pp. 34–50; Brian Tierney, *Medieval Poor Law:*

hospital as we conceive it today. This was not the case in the hospital of medieval Europe. The presence of monastic physicians in religious houses during the early Middle Ages makes it probable that the sick received some medical care. From the fourteenth century, secular physicians were increasingly associated with hospitals, to provide care for patients, but the physician was not yet an integral member of the hospital organization and remained independent.[12] Nevertheless, this initially loose association did provide the basis for another trend, which, from the seventeenth century on, led the medical profession increasingly to use the hospital for the study of disease and for its own practical education.

Economic, social, and political changes toward the end of the medieval period led, in the sixteenth century, to the replacement of the medieval institution by a hospital whose goals were not religious, but primarily social.[13] That is, the hospital, as it existed from the sixteenth century through the eighteenth century, was intended to help in the maintenance of social order by providing for the sick and the needy. It was an instrument of society to ameliorate suffering, to diminish poverty, to eradicate mendicity, and thus to help maintain public order, and it remained an institution that combined the care of the sick, an old-age home, an alms house, an orphanage, and in some instances a guest house. In its organization and opera-

---

A Sketch of Canonical Theory and Its Application in England (Berkeley: University of California Press, 1959), p. 87; Siegfried Reicke, *Das deutsche Spital und sein Recht im Mittelalter* (*Kirchenrechtliche Abhandlungen*) (Stuttgart, 1932).

[12] E. A. Hammond, "Physicians in Medieval English Religious Houses," *Bull. Hist. Med.* 35 (1961): 74–77; Werner Bubb, *Das Stadtarztamt zu Basel: Seine Entwicklungsgeschichte vom Jahre 1529 bis zur Gegenwart*, Basel dissertation (Zurich: Diss. Druckerei A.-G. Gebr. Leeman & Co., 1942), p. 11; A. F. La Cava, *Igiene e Sanità. Statuti di Milano del Sec.* XIV (Milan, 1946), pp. 40, 60–61, 71.

[13] Friedrich Paret, "Der Einfluss der Reformation auf die Armenpflege," *Zeitfragen des christlichen Volkslebens* 21 (1896): 46; F. R. Salter, ed., *Some Early Tracts on Poor Relief* (London: Methuen & Co., 1929); C. L. Steinbicker, *Poor Relief in the Sixteenth Century* (Washington, D.C.: Catholic University of America, 1937).

tion, the early modern hospital still retained various features of its predecessors. One of these was that medical care was a function of the hospital, but not its primary one.

During this period, however, various forces and developments external to the hospital eventually transformed it into what is now characteristic of economically developed countries. This hospital, the product of the industrial and scientific revolutions, may be called the health-workshop or medical-factory type. Here medical care is a primary goal of the institution and its provision is governed chiefly by scientific-technological norms and the requirements of organizational rationality and economy. Yet this hospital still retains features derived from its past that are not always congruent with its ostensible goals and norms. For this reason among others it is important to study the historical process by which an age-old institution has been transformed from a hostel for the sick poor into a medical center which we hope will eventually be available to all with health needs.

What I have just said applies in general also to medical education. All education presupposes some goal or ideal, and medical education is no exception. The purpose of a medical school is to turn out a physician who will come as close as possible to an ideal concept. However, it is also important to keep in mind that there are no absolute aims in medical education. Aims have changed and evolved in the course of time, and the process of change continues. The changing ideals, goals, or aims of medical education are a response to changing conditions in society and reflect the tasks assigned to the medical profession.

III

Since the end of the nineteenth century and to an increasing degree following the First World War, the physician and his practice have become inextricably intermixed with the increasingly complex organization which exists for the provision of medical care. This development is an aspect of the great social changes that have taken place in our society and mirrors a given state of societal evolution.

We have shifted from a rural to an urban society, from an agricultural to an industrial society, and we are continuing to move farther and farther in this direction.

In such a society, medicine and its practice will inevitably be different than it was in the past. For one thing, the range of scientific knowledge relevant to medicine has been immensely broadened in the last few generations. There has been a reduction of empiricism and an increasing endeavor to teach medicine on the basis of scientific principles. Hand in hand with these developments has come a more precise, more extensive, and more effective technology, together with a variety of organizational systems to operate it. As a result there is a growing need for a new physician to deal adequately with the health problems of such a social order. In the past, the healer was at various times a priest, a craftsman, a cleric, a medical jack-of-all-trades, and a scientist. Today, he must be not only scientifically trained in the physical and biological sciences, but also so oriented that he will be concerned with and knowledgeable about the place and functions of medicine in a highly organized, complex, industrial society.

In short, what I have been pointing to is that medicine, broadly speaking, must be viewed in its social context if we wish to understand what we are dealing with. Medicine represents a functional aspect of society and mirrors various social changes as they occur. On the other hand, by developments that may have far-reaching effects, it also affects the social context of which it is a part.

For example, many serious infectious diseases began to wane before the full impact of the bacteriological discoveries of the later nineteenth century made themselves felt. Beginning about 1870 there was a continuing downward trend in mortality due to a decline in the frequency of certain diseases, chiefly smallpox, typhoid and typhus fevers, tuberculosis, malaria, and yellow fever. The trend was roughly the same in most progressive areas, particularly the municipalities of western Europe and America, and undoubtedly reflects in part the impact of the earlier sanitary reform movement. On the theory that "a clean city is a healthy city," housing was improved, the physical environment was cleaned up, efforts were made to provide unadulterated food and clean water; in short, action was taken to provide decent living conditions. The English experience with typhus fever is an excellent case in point. Until 1870 there was very little variation in the death rate from "fever" in London. For the decade 1861 to 1870 the rate was 904 per million, but in the succeeding decade (1871 to 1880) it declined to 374. During this period, typhus fever was officially separated from other "fevers" and in the next two decades its decline was nothing short of spectacular. In 1906, three years before Nicolle's discovery that the body louse transmitted typhus, the annual report of the London County Council stated that there were no more deaths from the disease that year. Slum clearance, regulation of lodging houses, increased use of cotton clothing, especially underwear, and consequent improvement in personal cleanliness played their part in reducing the prevalence of typhus fever.

One result of the reduction of morbidity and mortality from the communicable diseases of infancy, childhood, and early adulthood is that people live longer and society must concern itself increasingly with the health problems of a maturing population. What this means in quantitative terms can be seen from the following figures. According to W. S. Thompson, the probable number of survivors to age 65 from 1,000 births in the United States increased from 325 in 1875 to 695 in 1940.[14] For Europe, an estimate by M. Pascua is illuminating. Based on the death rates of 1900, he calculated the number of deaths that would have occurred in Europe in 1947 and showed a theoretical saving of 1.75 million lives for that year. In 1900, only 13 million persons, or 18 per cent of the population of the United States, were in the "over 45" age group. Fifty years later this group comprised 43 million persons, or 30 per cent of the population. As a result, among the important medical problems that confront us today are the control of the chronic or degenerative con-

[14] W. S. Thompson, "The Demographic Revolution in the United States," *Ann. Amer. Acad. Pol. Soc. Sci.* (1949): 262–266; P. K. Whelpton, "A History of Population Growth in the United States," *Scientific Monthly* (1948): 67–86.

ditions—cancer, cardiovascular-renal conditions, arthritis, mental changes associated with aging, and musculo-skeletal diseases.

Clearly, we are at present more than ever aware that medicine is changing in terms of organization and modes of practice, and that it is branching out in new directions under the stimuli of demographic change, scientific and technologic development, and shifting social and economic conditions. This means that the responsibilities of the physician in the future will not be what they have been in the past. These changes require of the medical profession an understanding of the medical past in relation to the present, so that the future may be faced more clearly. For example, a considerable amount of useless talk about the plight of general practice and the family doctor might be eliminated if more physicians had some real knowledge of the historical evolution of the general practitioner. This is one of the important functions of medical history—to lay bare the origins of medical institutions, ideals, and values and to help explain their role and significance. The translation of medical and other values into health policy is historically conditioned, and the history of medicine can throw light on this aspect as well. But it is important, in endeavoring to understand the medical past and present, to remember that medicine is a social activity, undertaken within the context of human need and group life.

The Diseases of Civilization: Achievements and Illusions

RENÉ DUBOS, Ph.D.

The Rockefeller University, New York

THE AVERAGE EXPECTANCY OF LIFE has greatly increased in all the countries that have adopted the ways of life of Western civilization, but, surprising as it may seem, there has not been any significant increase in true longevity and we are as much as ever a disease-ridden society. I shall first attempt to clarify this paradox, then discuss the factors that are responsible for the fact that despite medical progress modern adults are neither longer lived nor healthier than adults were at the beginning of the century.

In the past, a very large percentage of children died during the first few years of life, usually before the age of five; this is still true in most parts of the world and in the underprivileged communities of the United States. In contrast, most children now survive into adulthood wherever social conditions are favorable. The practical elimination of the nutritional and infectious diseases that used to be responsible for childhood mortality accounts for all the increase in the average expectancy of life *at birth*.

Life expectancy past the age of forty-five, however, has remained much the same for many decades. Furthermore, it is not greater in countries or social groups that can afford elaborate medical care than in underprivileged communities. This is due to the great number of deaths caused by disorders of the vascular system, various forms of cancers, and in general the chronic and degenerative diseases which affect chiefly the adult population and for which there is no dependable method of prevention or cure.

It used to be thought that chronic and degenerative diseases had become more frequent simply because more people lived long enough to become victims. But this assumption is no longer tenable. The sad truth is that many aspects of the modern ways of life and of our environment constitute physiological stresses to which man cannot adapt successfully and which account for the increase in what one may call diseases of civilization. We are much in the dark concerning the precise etiological mechanisms of *chronic* and *degenerative* diseases, which now spoil the adult and later years of life; but there is no doubt that many of them are caused by environmental and social influences which affect most human beings in affluent societies. They are not inherent in man's nature, but are the consequences of his inadequate responses to conditions which differ drastically from those under which he evolved and to which he is still biologically and mentally adapted.

I

During the next few decades, most people in industrialized countries will live in large urban agglomerations. While there is no evidence that physical and mental health is inevitably impaired by urbanization and industrialization, the urban experience of mankind is so limited that a final judgment of the issue is not yet possible. Man has lived in cities, even in crowded ones, since neolithic times, but until recently the urban population was constantly being renovated by the influx of nonurban people migrating from primitive areas and rural environments. If present trends continue, however, the whole world will be urbanized and this biological transfusion will no longer be possible.

In the very near future most children of city dwellers will be born, will develop, and will have and raise their own children in urban environments. There is no way to foresee the biological and social consequences of urban life continued uninterruptedly for several generations.

Urban life exists in many different forms. One extreme is found in compact cities of continental Europe—Paris, Hamburg, Milan, or Athens—where most people live in apartments. Another extreme is found in the sprawling agglomerations of Los Angeles, Houston, and Sydney, where most people live in detached houses. But, granted that living in a compact city differs in many aspects from living in a sprawling agglomeration, all urban environments impose on human life certain common characteristics which are determined by technological forces.

If one were to judge from the physical appearance and behavior of people in westernized countries, it would seem that most human beings readily make a successful adjustment to the new ways of life created by urbanization and industrialization. Yet the demand for medical care and for hospital facilities is constantly increasing in all Western countries. One of the reasons for this increased demand is certainly that modern man has become more demanding with regard to health—and less willing than his ancestors to accept infirmities, pains, and blemishes. A more important reason, however, is that increasing numbers of persons suffer from chronic ailments—both physical and mental—which do not necessarily destroy life but ruin its later phases.

II

Although there is little precise knowledge of the mechanisms that relate environmental factors to chronic and degenerative diseases, it seems worthwhile to consider briefly some of the biological manifestations of the urban technological environment.

Gross malnutrition used to be common among urban dwellers in the past, but this is no longer the case in prosperous countries. The city dweller may even enjoy some nutritional advantage over the farmer, because the foodstuffs available to him are commonly more varied and fresher than those found in country stores.

Unfortunately, little is known of the kind of nutrition best suited to modern urban life. Nutritional requirements were determined two generations ago for vigorous and physically active young men. These requirements certainly do not fit automated, air-conditioned life. Much also remains to be learned concerning the needs of the mother during pregnancy and of her child during early postnatal life. Many pediatricians believe that the big baby is not necessarily a healthy baby. Too generous nutrition during early life may so affect the child that his nutritional demands remain excessively large thereafter—with undesirable physiological and behavioral consequences.

Infectious processes were among the most serious threats of city life in the past. Although the dangers to urban populations from this source have been decreased by public health practices and antibacterial drugs, their impact is still far greater than commonly assumed. On the other hand, it is possible that urban man develops resistance to certain infectious agents as a result of herd immunity. Influenza, for example, may never again achieve the catastrophic severity of the 1917–1918 epidemic, because most urban populations are highly mobile and consequently exposed at frequent intervals to the group of viruses responsible for this disease. The level of immunity acquired thereby may not be high enough to prevent reinfection completely, but sufficient nevertheless to protect against its most serious consequences.

Most forms of environmental pollution, including noise, are universal in industrialized countries and are often at their worst outside the city—for example, on heavily traveled highways or on bodies of water crowded with motorboats. Sewage, organic chemicals, and such mineral fertilizers as phosphates and nitrates pollute not only city reservoirs but also all natural waterways and lakes. Exhausts from motorcars, factories, and incinerators are incorporated into the smog that is almost as intense over suburbs as over compact cities and is progressively spreading over all the land.

No systematic studies have been made concerning the biological activities of the various kinds of air and water pollutants. Very little attention, for example, has been paid to the colloidal stuff released from automobile tires, or to the asbestos particles released from brake linings and from materials used for insulation by the building trade. Yet these particulate materials constitute a very large percentage of the total mass of air pollutants and are of a size that allows them to reach deep into the pulmonary tract. Since most kinds of environmental pollutants produced by modern technology did not reach significant levels until one or two decades ago, the worst effects of pollution are yet to be recognized.

Disturbances of biological rhythms resulting from modern ways of life may have deleterious effects on human health. Every person shifted from day to night duty or vice versa is aware of the difficulties resulting from hormonal misadjustments that such shifts entail. Similarly, every traveler has experienced the physiological discomfort associated with the rapid time change encountered when traveling by jet aircraft from one continent to another. Bright illumination late into the night and uniform temperature maintained throughout the year by air conditioning unquestionably contribute to comfort and efficiency. But it may turn out that these advantages will have to be paid for later in the form of pathological effects—yet to be determined because they have not been looked for. Grave pathological effects have been demonstrated in chickens exposed throughout the year to artificial light for increasing egg production and in frogs manipulated at different periods in their biological cycles. But hardly anything is known of the effects produced on man by disturbances of his normal physiological rhythms.

Along with environmental pollution and noise, crowding and its consequences are aspects of city life most commonly objected to. The fact is, however, that countless human beings appear to have elected to live among crowds throughout history—and even in prehistory. Rome, during the imperial period, the medieval fortified towns, and the cities of the Industrial Revolution all exhibited population densities that have not been exceeded in our own times. Modern cities are larger but generally less crowded than those of the past. Hong Kong and Holland are among the most crowded areas of the world, yet their populations enjoy good physical and mental health because they have slowly developed in the course of centuries patterns of human relationships that minimize social conflicts and allow persons to retain their identity and a large measure of individual freedom. This does not mean that man can indefinitely increase the density of his populations, but only that the safe limits have not been determined.

III

One difficulty in the etiological analysis of the diseases of civilization is that many changes in the surroundings and ways of life occur simultaneously and so rapidly that their individual pathological effects cannot be determined. Furthermore, change per se often acts as a pathological agent, irrespective of the nature of the conditions that are changed.

In many cases, for example, the deleterious effects of crowding result not so much from high population density as from the social disturbances associated with sudden increase in density. The appalling amount of biological and mental disease during the Industrial Revolution had several different causes, but one of the most important was certainly the fact that immense numbers of people from rural areas had to live and function in the densely populated tenements and industrial settlements of the mushrooming cities before they had had time to make physiological and emotional adaptation to their new way of life. Yet it took but a few decades to convert these rural populations into urban ones for whom high population density became almost a pleasant state of affairs. In contrast, there is some indication that rapid decrease in population density, as is occurring at present in the Great Plains of North America, may increase the incidence of mental disorders. The rapid mobility of populations from one area to another is also contributing at present to the patterns of diseases in technological societies.

The history of mankind demonstrates that most human beings can make biological and social adjustments that enable them to adapt and continue to function effectively even under extremely stressful conditions. However, while the phrase "adaptive response" conveniently describes the interplay between man and his environment, the concepts of adaptation developed by biologists are not entirely suitable to the analysis of human medical problems.

The general biologist usually defines the word *adaptation* in Darwinian terms. For him the word implies a state of fitness to a given environment, enabling the species to multiply and to invade new territories. In this light, man is remarkably adapted to life in highly urbanized and industrialized societies, as shown by the fact that his populations continuously increase and that he spreads urbanization and industrialization to more and more of the earth. It is obvious, on the other hand, that further population increase has become objectionable and may soon become catastrophic. In applying the concept of adaptation to man it is therefore necessary to use criteria different from those used in general biology.

Physiologists or psychologists give to the word *adaptation* a meaning different from that implied in Darwinian population theory. But their interpretation also fails to take into account the peculiarities of human life. For physiologists and psychologists, a response is adaptive when it enables the person to maintain homeostasis through metabolic, hormonal, or mental processes that tend to correct the disturbing effects environmental forces exert on the body and the mind. Such adaptive responses contribute to the welfare of the organism at the time they occur, but unfortunately they often have secondary effects that are deleterious at a later date. When evaluated over man's whole life span, homeostatic mechanisms are less successful than commonly assumed, because many, if not most, chronic disorders are the secondary and delayed consequences of adaptive responses that were useful at first but are faulty in the long run.

It has long been recognized, of course, that homeostatic mechanisms can lead to unhomeostatic effects, particularly when the homeostatic response is excessive. In traumatic shock, for example, intense vasoconstriction is homeostatic to the extent that it preserves blood pressure, but it is unhomeostatic at the same time because it deprives organs and tissues, such as the kidney, of their vital blood flow. In the hypervolemia of heart failure the congestive state is useful up to a point in filling a weakened heart chamber, but it leads ultimately to total failure by way of excessive vascular pressures and overdilated heart chambers. The inflammatory reaction helps in fixing or destroying the aggressive agent, but it can in many ways destroy the organ while attempting to protect the body.

Most important, as already mentioned, is the fact that homeostatic mechanisms commonly have delayed and indirect consequences responsible for the pathology of many chronic disorders. The production of scar tissue is a homeostatic response because it heals wounds and helps to check the spread of infection. But fibrosis in the liver or in the kidney means cirrhosis or glomerular nephritis; scar tissue may freeze the joints in rheumatoid arthritis or may choke the breathing process in the lungs.

Many other examples readily suggest themselves, among them the various forms of hyperimmune responses and such so-called compensatory reactions as compensating polycythemia or compensating emphysema. These processes exert a protective or reparative function when they first occur, but they can become destructive in the long run. All too often the wisdom of the body is a very shortsighted wisdom.

Atmospheric pollution provides striking examples both of man's ability to function in a biologically undesirable environment and of the dangers inherent in this adaptability. Ever since the beginning of the Industrial Revolution the inhabitants of northern Europe have been heavily exposed to many types of air pollutants produced by incomplete combustion and the fumes from chemical plants; such exposure is rendered even more objectionable by the inclemency of the Atlantic climate. Long experience with pollution and bad weather has resulted in the development of physiological reactions and of living habits which have adaptive value, as proved by the fact that northern Europeans accept most cheerfully their dismal environment. Such adaptive responses to pollution occur all over the world in the heavily industrialized areas, where people function effectively despite the almost constant presence of irritating substances in the air they breathe.

Unfortunately, the respiratory tract continuously registers the insult of the various air pollutants, even among persons who seem almost unaware of the smog surrounding them. As a result, chronic pulmonary disease now constitutes the greatest single medical problem in northern Europe. It is increasing in prevalence at an alarming rate also in North America, and it will probably spread to all areas undergoing industrialization. There is evidence, furthermore, that air pollution increases the incidence of various types of cancers as well as the numbers of fatalities among persons suffering from vascular diseases. But the long and indefinite span of time between cause and effect makes it difficult to establish convincingly the etiological relationships.

The delayed effects of air pollutants constitute models for the kind of medical problems likely to arise in the future from other forms of environmental pollution. Wherever convenient, chemical pollution of air, water, and food will be sufficiently controlled to prevent the kind of toxic effects that are immediately disabling and otherwise obvious. Human beings will then tolerate without complaint concentrations of environmental pollutants that do not constitute such a serious nuisance as to interfere with social and economic life. But continued exposure to low levels of toxic agents will eventually result in a great variety of delayed pathological manifestations that will not be detected at the time of exposure, and may not become evident until several decades later.

Adjustment to the various forms of malnutrition also has distant consequences of far-reaching importance. For example, persons who have been born and raised in an environment where food intake is quantitatively or qualitatively inadequate seem to achieve a physiological adaptation to the kind of malnutrition that they have experienced in youth. Such adaptation, however, creates a vicious cycle of metabolic difficulties and mental retardation or indolence. Similarly, children whose diets are excessively abundant and rich tend as adults to become large eaters and thus may become more prone to vascular diseases.

As a result of the erroneous belief that microbial diseases have been "conquered," there is a tendency to regard the so-called minor infections as inconsequential problems. Yet these ailments erode the functional integrity of the body, progressively damaging the respiratory, digestive, and urinary tracts, as well as the kidneys, and perhaps also the blood vessels. Like other stresses to which man becomes adjusted, minor infectious processes probably play a part in the diseases of the modern world.

Man is a gregarious animal; he generally tends to accept crowded environments and even to seek them. Constant and intimate contact with hordes of human beings has come to constitute the "normal" way of life. This change has certainly brought about all kinds of phenotypic adaptations to social environments that constituted biological and emotional threats in the past. But the long-range consequences of this adaptation are not known. If constant and extreme crowding has pathological effects, these will have an insidious course, their expressions being determined not so much by the initial effect of the stimulus on a particular target organ as by the complex secondary responses evoked from the whole organism and from the whole social group.

IV

The responses to environmental stimuli made by the organism during the very early phases of its development, including the intrauterine phase, deserve special emphasis because they exert profound and lasting effects on the physical, physiological, and behavioral characteristics of the adult. Often, indeed, such effects appear irreversible.

The following are a few of the many observations made in laboratory animals which exemplify the remote and indirect manifestations of early influences:

> A single exposure of young female mice to a small dose of radiation (25 R) does not destroy their fertility, but it shortens their reproductive life span—by inactivating some of their oocytes in immature follicle stages. Since a long-delayed effect on fertility can thus be traced to oocyte damage occurring twenty-four hours after irradiation, there is reason to believe that other complex late effects may also be the indirect consequences of other types of cell death occurring immediately following radiation.

A single injection into neonatal mice of particulate pollutants common in urban air produced a high incidence of hepatomas much later during the adult life of the treated animals.

Subclinical infections contracted at birth and mild nutritional deficiencies during gestation or lactation have been found to depress the growth rate and adult size in various animal species, even if the subsequent conditions were optimum for adult development. Many different types of stimuli that impinge on the organism during its early formative stages (even *in utero*) can likewise affect the learning ability and behavioral patterns of the adult.

V

The greatest improvements in health have been achieved by eliminating the most obvious agencies of disease, rather than by treating their pathological manifestations. The following changes have probably been among the most influential in this respect: sanitary measures against the spread of gastrointestinal infections; vaccination against smallpox, diphtheria, and a few other infectious diseases; the social practices that brought about a spectacular fall in mortality of tuberculosis long before vaccination or any of the antituberculous drugs were available; better food, clothing, housing, and working conditions; less exacting physical work; and more effective protection against inclemencies of the weather.

Many of the beneficial factors mentioned above correspond to what is generally referred to as "higher living standards." There is no doubt that higher living standards have rendered the population more resistant to various infections and other stresses. But there is reason to fear that we have now reached a phase of diminishing returns in this regard. In fact, the high level of prosperity is creating a new set of medical problems. Environmental pollution, excessive food intake, lack of physical exercise, the constant bombardment of stimuli, and the estrangement of civilized life from the natural biological rhythms are among the many consequences of urbanized and industrialized life that have direct or indirect pathological effects. In brief, it can no longer be taken for granted that a further rise in living standards will result in health improvement. The more probable situation is that it will result in a new pattern of diseases.

Even if we succeed in identifying the factors that are responsible for the increase in chronic and degenerative diseases, it will prove extremely difficult to control them, because all aspects of the urban and industrial environment are so intimately interwoven in the social fabric. Other difficulties have their origin in individual attitudes. Keeping streets and houses clear of refuse, filtering and chlorinating the water supplies, watching over the purity of food products, assuring a safe minimum of air in public places constitute measures that can be applied by the collectivity in an anonymous manner, so to speak, and without interfering seriously with individual freedom. These measures do not demand personal effort from their beneficiaries and are therefore readily accepted.

In contrast, any measure that requires individual discipline and effort is likely to be neglected. Almost everybody is aware of the dangers associated with overeating, with failure to engage in physical exercise, with chain cigarette-smoking, with constant exposure to polluted environments and to social stimuli, and with excessive consumption of alcohol and other stimulants or depressants. But few persons are willing to make the individual effort that would be required to avoid these dangers. Furthermore, the consequences of environmental threats are so often indirect and delayed that the public is hardly aware of them.

VI

The mass diseases of the past were fairly directly connected with the natural environment. In contrast, the chronic and degenerative conditions, as well as the mental disorders, which constitute the mass diseases of today in prosperous countries, are integrated in a much more complex manner with the ways of life and the socio-cultural environment. For this reason they are much less amenable to community-based control than are the nutritional and infectious diseases and they demand greater emphasis on the cooperation and interest of the individual. Hence, we are faced with a need to reformulate medical policies in such a manner that the conventional public health practices that emerged from nineteenth-century science will be supplemented by more personal relationships between physician and patient.

The physicians and medical scientists of the late nineteenth and early twentieth centuries proceeded on the assumption that most disease problems originate from poverty and filth and therefore can be solved by improving living conditions. This hypothesis placed the war against microbes and malnutrition at the center of the medical stage. The dramatic fall in mortality rates all over the Western world leaves no doubt as to the efficacy of the attack against the infectious and nutritional diseases which dominated the medical picture after the first Industrial Revolution.

Around the turn of the century the focus of medical interest shifted from the environment to the intimate structures and mechanisms of living organisms. Studies on the spread of infection or of the quality of foodstuffs lost ground to the chemical analysis of immunological processes, of intermediary metabolism, or of endocrine control. Even the Pavlovian reflexes and Freudian complexes are beginning to appear old-fashioned when compared with the detailed analysis of neural mechanisms or of memory storage and retrieval.

This change of scientific focus has had large practical consequences. Whereas the greatest contributions to health during the nineteenth century were in the prevention of disease through manipulation of the environment, the most brilliant successes of twentieth-century medicine have been in the treatment of disease through action on the intimate mechanisms of the body. The twentieth century can of course boast of spectacular feats in the prevention of disease, but these achievements have come in all cases from the direct application of nineteenth-century concepts. For example, the development of new vaccines against bacterial and viral infections did not depend on knowledge of body structures or functions. The twentieth-century achievements in immunization were the fruits of theoretical concepts developed and successfully used by nineteenth-century immunologists. Similarly, the virtual elimination of deficiency diseases was achieved through nutritional improvements which were little influenced by knowledge of the precise role played by vitamins or amino acids in metabolic, synthetic, or regulatory processes. On the other hand, the use of insulin and other hormones, the dietary control of phenylketonuria, the maintenance of normal physiological processes during surgical interventions, the operation of artificial kidneys or of cardiac pacesetters are but a few examples of therapeutic procedures which could not have been developed without a detailed knowledge of body components and functions. There is even hope that some of the mental disorders can be managed through this approach.

The description of the organism in terms of its elementary structures and mechanisms and the doctrine of specific etiology have led to such spectacular achievements, both theoretical and practical, that, to create a medical utopia, it would seem sufficient to let medicine continue along the road on which it is now traveling. Yet there are signs that a change in direction is necessary, and indeed is about to be made.

The disorders of the body and of the mind are to a very large extent the consequences of inadequate responses to the environment. They involve not only a particular organ but the organism as a whole. For this reason, the practice of medicine demands of the physician a holistic attitude that goes beyond that of the experimental scientist.

Of special importance is the fact that the patient's responses are conditioned by past influences, especially the influences exerted by the factors which affected his early development. One of the greatest contributions of the Hippocratic school—and in our own times of Freud—has been to emphasize the importance of taking a "history" in the examination of the patient. History-taking will certainly become an even more important aspect of medical care in the future, when more is known of the extent to which the experiential past can affect all aspects of life, including resistance to disease.

Emergence of the Hospital as a Social Institution

JOHN H. KNOWLES, M.D.
General Director, The Massachusetts General Hospital, Boston
Professor of Medicine, Harvard University Medical School

THE HOSPITAL HAS EMERGED from its origins as a passive receptacle for the sick poor to the modern, acute, curative, highly technical "health center." We are now entering the third and most important stage in its evolution, which will see the centripetal forces of science and technology of the past half century matched by the centrifugal forces of social need. These forces will actively extend the hospital staff's influence out into the community to prevent disease and to research a system of medical care with the aims of reaching more people through improved accessibility and health education, and of containing costs through the better use of scarce health manpower and the use of lower-cost facilities where appropriate. Medicine, its institutions, and its people will then take their rightful place among the community's institutions, and the hospital will, in fact, become the "health center." Rational systematization of medical care is not incompatible with, nor need it interfere with improving the personal element of care, maintaining the private practice of medicine or the voluntary nature of our nation's best hospitals, or encouraging our precious pluralism. More positively, the preservation and improvement of all three elements are vital to the future of this country, regardless of professional interest.

The contemporary hospital has reached a unique position as a social instrument of society in its eternal battle with disease and suffering. Its present form has been shaped by the needs, as well as by the beliefs, values, and attitudes of society. The hospital is a mirror of society, reflecting not only its culture but also its economy. In just the past half century, science has contributed so heavily to the knowledge, treatment, and prevention of disease that the present science and technology of medicine can no longer be mastered by the individual. The resultant specialization in all areas of medicine and the massive technology contained within the walls of the urban teaching hospital have been of pronounced benefit to mankind. The steadily mounting benefits have created the social problem of rising expectations in a rapidly expanding, longer-lived population, progressively less able, individually, to afford the steadily rising cost of medical care.

The problems of medicine and hospitals today demand a more effective social technology for their solution. Society's potency increases with the increasing division of labor, while the individual's potency decreases. In the case of the hospital, social action by the total institution becomes mandatory if effective solutions of some of the social, political, and economic problems of medicine are to be found. A strong institutional social conscience leads to social action for the benefit of the community. As Titmuss has said, ". . . progress in medical science in psychological theories and in the specialized division of medical skill has converted medicine from an individual intuitive enterprise into a social service."[1]

Historical Perspective

The earliest hospitals were the healing temples of ancient Egypt, the public hospitals of Buddhist India and the Mohammedan East, and the sick houses (Beth Holem) of Israel. The earliest physician was both priest and magician. Disease represented the work of evil spirits and could be induced by infractions of religious codes. The

[1] R. M. Titmuss, *Essays on the Welfare State* (New Haven: Yale University Press, 1959), p. 135.

ancient Oriental custom of hospitality for guests and travelers pervaded the Levant and houses were built where weary travelers and strangers could stop for food and lodging and, if sick, nursing care. The very derivation of the word *hospital* shows what an important part these travelers and their hosts played in the evolution of the hospital. *Hospital* comes from the Latin, *hospes*, meaning host or guest. The English word *hospital* comes from the Old French *hospitale* as do the words *hostel* and *hotel*. All were originally derived from the Latin. These three words, *hospital*, *hostel*, and *hotel*, although of different meaning today, were at one time used interchangeably.

It was the prototype of the British voluntary teaching hospitals of London that ultimately arose in America, but only after more than a century following the first settlements. As Shryock has noted, "In Spanish and French colonies the church set up such institutions more promptly. But the Anglican and non-conformist English churches had given up the hospital tradition and state or 'voluntary' agencies acted only under the cumulative pressures of public need, secular humanitarianism, and professional initiative."[2]

In discussing the evolution of institutions that housed the sick, I shall confine my comments to the Massachusetts Bay Colony and Boston, particularly the university-affiliated teaching hospital and primarily the Massachusetts General Hospital (M.G.H.). Of the roughly 7,000 hospitals that exist in the United States today, there are 140 with university affiliation, 1,000 accredited as teaching institutions, and over 5,000 which are not classified or accredited as teaching institutions. It should also be noted that we are a nation of small hospitals (under 200 beds) and not large ones.

The most powerful stimulus to the founding of the American hospital was the process of urbanization as, indeed, the history of the city is the history of social progress (or social decline) in any civilization. Urbanization concentrated the need for care in a small area and provided the tools for the solution of the problems. Public health measures for the segregation of infectious disease in quaran-

[2] R. H. Shryock, *Medicine and Society in America: 1660–1860* (New York: New York University Press, 1960), p. 9.

tine hospitals very early fell under the jurisdiction of the General Court of Massachusetts, establishing the state's responsibility in these matters. The city produced the merchant prince with the social conscience who was to devote his fortune to private philanthropic work for the good of his fellow man. Intellectual activity abounded and flourished in the city. Educational institutions were founded and, finally, schools of medicine which needed institutions where teaching and learning could be by first hand experience.

Urbanization

The progressive urbanization of Boston was slow, initially, and gained rapidly only with the arrival of the nineteenth century. The population grew from 4,500 to 1680 to 11,000 in 1720[3] and to 32,896 in 1810.[4] As late as 1845 "Boston remained . . . a town of small traders, of petty artisans and handicraftsmen, and of great merchant princes who built fortunes out of their 'enterprise, intelligence, and frugality.' "[5] The merchant princes amassed their fortunes from entrepreneurial traffic between Boston, Oregon, and Canton; Southern ports and Liverpool; the West Indies and Russia. The town lacked a fertile back country, had no large source of labor, and lacked the power of a good water supply. Entrepreneurial activity was the only answer. The resultant wealth was wisely invested, and Boston became a great center of finance and banking, supplying the money for the first railroads in this country and gaining a firm hold on the development of the textile and shoe industries in Massachusetts. The home town of the merchant prince and the petty artisan contained favorable social conditions, and in 1790 it was said that poverty and pauperism were declining, relative to the total population.[6] And well they might, for "Boston offered few opportunities to those who lacked the twin advantages of birth and capi-

[3] L. Shattuck, *Census of Boston for the Year 1845* (City of Boston, 1846), p. 5.

[4] O. Handlin, *Boston's Immigrants* (Cambridge: Harvard University Press, 1959), p. 239.

[5] *Ibid.*, p. 11.

[6] Shattuck, *Census of Boston for the Year 1845*, p. 113.

tal."[7] Most immigrants, until the Irish hegira of the 1840's, passed through Boston on their way West or went directly to Philadelphia or New York.

Institutions for the Care of the Sick

What was the state of the public's health during this time and what were the provisions for the care of the sick? The original Colonial practice of "outdoor relief" whereby local citizens were paid to take the sick into their homes was soon outmoded as the burden increased and infectious diseases became the main public health problem.

Smallpox was the chief public health problem of the seventeenth and eighteenth centuries. Major epidemics hit Boston at least four times between 1644 and 1689 and seven times in the eighteenth century, beginning in 1721, with the last great epidemic occurring in 1792. The General Court had taken measures in 1699 and 1700 to provide for the isolation of townsfolk and quarantine of ships' crews known to have "the plague, smallpox, pestilential or malignant fever, or other contagious sickness, the infection whereof may probably be communicated to others."[8] An earlier "pesthouse" was replaced by the quarantine hospital built on Spectacle Island by the order of the General Court in 1717. Managed by the Town Selectmen, it was later abandoned and replaced in 1737 by one on Rainsford Island.

Some idea of the seriousness and magnitude of the smallpox epidemics can be gained from the figures in 1721 when the disease was introduced by the infected crew of a British ship newly arrived from the West Indies. Of the total population of 10,700 in the town, 5,759 contracted the disease and 842 or nearly 8 per cent of the total population, died. It was during this epidemic that Cotton Mather wrote to Dr. Zabdiel Boylston, urging him to try the inoculation method developed by Timoni of Constantinople. Subsequently, Dr. Boylston inoculated 242 persons in nearby towns and there were

[7] Handlin, *Boston's Immigrants*, p. 12.

[8] J. B. Blake, *Public Health in the Town of Boston, 1630–1822* (Cambridge: Harvard University Press, 1959), p. 33.

only six deaths. After much prolonged controversy, hospitals for inoculation and segregation of infected patients were approved and set up by the General Court as well as by private physicians, between 1764 and 1790. Dr. William Aspinwall's, which had 150 beds, was referred to as the "Grand Inoculation Hospital." Games, music, and parades were arranged for the patients. The inoculation hospital disappeared when Prof. Benjamin Waterhouse introduced Jennerian vaccination.

The first almshouse in Boston opened its doors in 1665. It was consumed by fire and a new one was built in 1686, which by 1790 had 300 occupants.[9] A bridewell for the disorderly and the insane, built in the early 1700's, and a workhouse for the able-bodied ne'er-do-wells, built in 1735, were immediately adjacent. It was stated that "earlier almshouses of Massachusetts were indicative of all that is evil in the eyes of social services. They admitted of slight if any separation of the sexes. They afforded no classification according to age. They housed little children with the prostitute, the vagrant, the drunkard, the idiot, and the maniac . . . they were schools for crime —breeders of immorality and chronic pauperism"[10] and, I might add, for the easy transmission of infectious disease among the impoverished sick.

In 1800, a new almshouse, designed by Charles Bulfinch, was built on the north side of Leverett Street in the West End, which was to stand until 1825. The Reverend John Bartlett was its chaplain, a fortunate assignment, as we shall see.

Meanwhile another institution, the forerunner of the present-day ambulatory medical clinic, was established through the efforts of the Massachusetts Humane Society, which had been founded in 1780. The Boston Dispensary was founded in 1796 for two reasons: (1) so that the sick could be cared for in their own houses and (2) so that they could be assisted at less expense to the public than in a hos-

[9] R. M. Lawrence, *Old Park Street and Its Vicinity* (Boston: Houghton Mifflin Co., 1922), pp. 33–35.

[10] R. W. Kelso, *The History of Public Poor Relief in Massachusetts* (Boston: Houghton Mifflin Co., 1922), p. 112.

pital or the almshouse.[11] Although described as a drug store with a physician for ambulatory patients, it served both the humanitarian and the economical reasons for its existence.[12]

Another institution for care of the sick was established at the turn of the nineteenth century. Agitation for construction of a hospital had been voiced by the Boston Marine Society at their meeting in October 1790. Its purpose was to care for merchant mariners, frequently far from home, in places where most medical care was being given for those fortunate enough to avoid the "pesthouses." A Congressional Bill entitled, "An Act for the Relief of Sick and Disabled Seamen" was signed by President John Adams on July 16, 1798, and established a form of compulsory, government-supervised sickness and accident insurance to provide medical care and hospitalization for seamen by the collection of twenty cents per month per mariner on every American merchant ship coming from a foreign port.[13] In 1803 a marine hospital was completed in Charlestown for the port of Boston, and in 1804 staff and patients moved to the new quarters from a temporary location set up in 1799 in the barracks buildings at Fort Independence on Castle Island. The new hospital housed an average of thirty patients.

The Medical Profession and Medical Education

The medical profession and the founding of the Harvard Medical School in 1782 played a crucial role in the founding of the M.G.H. With the English middle classes who first migrated to America came the first physicians—"ships' surgeons" or apprentices from London hospitals—not English physicians who enjoyed high social prestige and good incomes in London. Most of the early practitioners were peripatetic surgeon-apothecaries and, commonly, ministers doubling as physicians. Medical education consisted of the inden-

[11] W. R. Lawrence, *History of the Boston Dispensary* (Boston, 1859), p. 14.

[12] M. D. Davis and A. R. Warner, *Dispensaries: Their Management and Development* (New York: Macmillan Co., 1918), p. 6.

[13] J. W. Trask, *The United States Marine Hospital, Port of Boston* (Washington, D.C.: U.S. Public Health Service, 1940), pp. 11–12.

tured apprentice system. On the eve of the American Revolution, only 5 per cent of the 3,500 established medical practitioners held degrees. Scarcely 10 per cent had had any formal training.[14] Harvard College, founded in 1636 on a strongly puritanical and theological basis, had minister-physicians as its first two presidents. Its second and third presidents were graduates in medicine of Cambridge, England. By 1700, twenty-six graduates of Harvard College were said to have practiced medicine in New England, though none had a medical degree.[15] The indentured apprentice system remained the main form of medical education.

In 1773 Dr. Ezekiel Hersey left £1,000 to Harvard College to support a resident professor of anatomy and surgery. Edward A. Holyoke of Salem, a 1746 graduate of Harvard College, had among his many apprentices John Warren. On September 19, 1782, the Harvard Corporation adopted some twenty-two articles, probably authored by John Warren, which established the Harvard Medical School. Its first three professors were John Warren in anatomy and surgery, Benjamin Waterhouse in physic, and Aaron Dexter in chemistry and materia medica. The first lectures were delivered in the fall of 1784.

This new method of teaching was not universally applauded, as is shown by several public clashes of the Massachusetts Medical Society with the new medical school in Cambridge. The Society, founded in 1781, demanded the right to examine and license all physicians,[16] prevented use of the Boston Almshouse for the teaching of medical students, and defeated the Harvard Corporation's Proposal to the General Court for the establishment of a "public infirmary" in Cambridge for the care of the sick and the teaching of medical students.[17] The Boston Medical Society wrote that "the scheme of annexing a

14 Shryock, *Medicine and Society in America*, pp. 7–9.

15 H. R. Viets, *A Brief History of Medicine in Massachusetts* (Boston: Houghton Mifflin Co., 1930), p. 42.

16 T. E. Moore, "The Early Years of the Harvard Medical School," *Bull. Hist. Med.* 27 (1953): 530–561; esp. 535.

17 *Ibid.*, p. 555.

Medical Establishment in this Town to the College in Cambridge is not only impractical but nugatory."[18]

In 1782 Dr. Warren had been appointed to care for the sick in the almshouse. Although he took his apprentices there, not until 1810 were Harvard medical students allowed to enter the new almshouse for clinical training. At this time the almshouse had approximately 350 occupants, of whom about 50 were sick and infirm. Medical education at Harvard consisted of two winters of lectures and a third year as apprentice to a practitioner before a student could qualify for his degree in medicine. In 1807 Professor Benjamin Waterhouse, as chief physician of the new Boston Marine Hospital, urged that his institution be used for teaching medical students. In 1810 the medical school moved from Cambridge to Boston, and in 1816 it moved again. In 1847 it moved to quarters adjacent to the Massachusetts General Hospital and thirty-six years later to quarters almost equidistant from the M.G.H. and the rapidly growing Boston City Hospital. This hospital opened its doors in 1864 to meet the growing needs of a rapidly expanding immigrant population driven from Ireland by the great potato famines.

The Founding of the M.G.H.

I have attempted to describe various factors that were to result in the founding of the Massachusetts General Hospital in 1811: the development of the humanitarian spirit; the age of individualism; the advent of the merchant prince with a social conscience; the process of urbanization; the relative inadequacy of existing institutions for the care of the sick; and finally, the rise of the enquiring medical mind, scientific thought, and new concern for improving medical education, requiring that a hospital be available for teaching.

The well-to-do were cared for at home—a situation that prevailed until the early years of the twentieth century. Philadelphia and New York had already established hospitals in almost identical circum-

[18] T. F. Harrington, *The Harvard Medical School: A History, Narrative and Documentary* (New York, 1905), pp. 274–278.

stances. The Boston philanthropists and doctors were anxious that such a humanitarian institution grace their city.

All the factors and forces for the creation of such an institution were present. The Reverend John Bartlett, chaplain of the Boston Almshouse, was spurred on by the Christian ethic and the inhumane conditions of the almshouse. James Jackson and John Collins Warren represented the medical profession and the need for medical education. Merchant princes were represented by John Phillips and Peter Brooks.[19] The letter from Warren and Jackson to the wealthy and influential citizens of Boston, and the subsequent report of the legislative committee recommending the state's approval of the hospital's charter summarize beautifully the social need for such an institution, the responsibility with which it would be charged. The report stated: "The Hospital, thus established, is intended to be a receptacle for patients from all parts of the Commonwealth, afflicted with diseases of a peculiar nature, requiring the most skillful treatment, and presenting cases for instruction in the study and practice of surgery and physic.

"Among the unfortunate objects of this charitable project, particular provision is to be made for such as the wisdom of Providence may have seen fit to visit with the most terrible of all human maladies—a deprivation of reason. . . .[20]

On February 25, 1811, the General Court granted to James Bowdoin and fifty-five other prominent Bostonians a charter for the incorporation of the Massachusetts General Hospital. Active interest and participation by the state in the conduct and maintenance of the hospital was assured from the outset, not only through repeated financial aid, but also through the practice which continues to this day: the governor's appointment of four of the twelve trustees.

By 1817 enough private money was available so that, with final aid from the state in the form of prison labor and granite, construction could begin. Charles Bulfinch was the architect. James Jackson

[19] L. K. Eaton, *New England Hospitals: 1790–1833* (Ann Arbor: University of Michigan Press, 1957), pp. 34–36.

[20] As quoted in J. E. Garland, *Every Man Our Neighbor* (Boston: Little, Brown and Co., 1961), p. 5.

was appointed physician and John C. Warren surgeon for the M.G.H. On September 3, 1821, the first patient was admitted. No other application was made until September 20.[21] The first *Annual Report*, printed in 1822, contained what today would be considered direct advertising, beginning, "We entreat all those into whose hands this address may fall, to reflect well upon the advantages which this Institution offers . . ." It then listed the comforts and advantages of hospital care.[22] The public was slow to forget experiences in the pesthouse and almshouse, and as late as 1849 the hospital was not yet completely filled.[23]

By 1823 there were ninety-three beds, and in 1824 the Trustees ordered that medical students and doctors attending operations should be admitted free and not charged by the staff.

In the early years—as today—the most pressing problem was the gap between the cost of running the hospital and the income from patients, friends, and endowment. The idea of free-bed subscription was instituted by the Massachusetts Humane Society in 1824, giving the hospital enough money to support six free beds for five years. Subsequent annual drives were conducted seeking support of free beds, and in 1826 "23 beds were occupied . . . at an average expense of $3.52 per week for an average stay of 5½ weeks."[24]

At the turn of this century a leaflet describing the work of the Massachusetts General Hospital read in part: "The Massachusetts General Hospital is a private institution, supported solely by voluntary contributions and the receipts from those patients who pay board . . ." After describing the types of application for admission, the statement continued: "Contagious cases are not admitted to the hospital, and only such chronic cases as can be partially relieved by temporary treatment. Regular charges to paying patients are as follows: In the Jackson Ward (private) $35 per week; in the Bigelow

[21] N. I. Bowditch, *History of the Massachusetts General Hospital* (Boston, 1851), p. 5.

[22] *Address of the Trustees of the Massachusetts General Hospital to the Subscribers and to the Public* (Boston, 1822), p. 16.

[23] *M.G.H. Annual Report, 1849*, p. 5.

[24] Eaton, *New England Hospitals*, p. 105.

Ward \$21 per week; in small rooms in the Townsend in the General Wards \$10.50 per week. The outpatient department is for the poor only and is open between 9 and 10 in the morning, Sundays and holidays excepted."

Today a similar flyer would read:

> The Massachusetts General Hospital is a part private, part public institution—supported by (1) voluntary contributions and endowment income; (2) involuntary payments by overcharged private patients; (3) state and federal funds under the Social Security Act of 1935 and the amendments of 1966, Medicare and Medicaid; (4) the reimbursements of Blue Cross and commercial insurance companies; (5) the payments of a steadily diminishing number of direct-paying patients; and (6) progressively smaller amounts of money from the United Fund. Contagious cases, including tuberculosis are admitted to the hospital, and chronic cases are accepted for rehabilitation as well as help with their ultimate disposition to the necessary chronic care facilities. Regular charges to paying patients, third-party payers such as the Blue Cross and to state welfare departments are (when appropriate) \$560 per week in a private room, \$434 in a semiprivate room, and \$385 in a ward room. The outpatient department is for all social and economic classes and is open 7 days a week (in conjunction with the Emergency Ward), 24 hours a day, including all holidays. . . .

Comparison of these two statements shows a change in character and function of the hospital, evolving from a totally voluntary, low-cost, passive receptacle for the indigent sick to a quasi-voluntary, high-cost, positive force for all social and economic classes. It is now called, euphemistically, the "health center." The three major revolutions affecting medicine in the past half century—expansion of medical knowledge through science, development of social welfare programs, including the various forms of prepayment for medical care, and establishment of the present form of medical education—have made today's hospital what it is and what it is not. Medical science is well established, its triumphs are legion. The social and economic programs and problems of medicine remain largely unstudied and unknown in most medical schools. I shall return to this theme later.

Three Contributions of the Hospital as a Social Instrument

I would like to indicate three examples of the hospital's role as a social instrument, examples of the institutional effort to fulfill the needs of the community through the function of patient care.

Social Service

The prime example of an institutional social conscience arose in 1905, after Dr. Richard Cabot had been appointed physician to the M.G.H. Out-Patient Department. As Washburn stated:

> From its very earliest days, the General Hospital has shown an interest in its patients' problems and a humane attempt to lighten their burdens. When the Hospital was a small affair, the Trustees themselves visited the patients regularly. In many instances they saw to it that relief over and above medical care was provided. As doctors and patients and Hospital officers were a small family, the troubles of the patients and the underlying causes of their disease, their disposition upon discharge were considered, and often remedied and alleviated. . . . the Resident Physician (Director) or his assistant took great pains to see to it that discharged patients were properly escorted to their homes, that patients left on the doorstep were suitably placed, and that allied administrative problems were handled as humanely and efficiently as the means and facilities at their disposal would permit. The problems were not so difficult when New England had a homogeneous, uncrowded population, with a good standard of living.
>
> With the tremendous unrestricted immigration of the latter part of the 19th and the early part of the 20th century, the difficulties became greater and more complex.[25]

It was Dr. Richard Cabot who recognized the need for a more coordinated, formalized program of social help when he employed two full-time workers in 1905. The workers' sole function was service for problems relating to the care of the patient. Their 1906 report listed work which included courses in hygiene, infant feeding and care, "vacations and country outings" where it seemed a neces-

[25] F. A. Washburn, *The Massachusetts General Hospital: Its Development 1900–1935* (Boston: Houghton Mifflin Co., 1939), p. 459.

sary part of treatment, help in finding jobs or changing jobs according to the medical need, provision for patients "dumped" at the hospital, and "assistance to patients needing treatment after discharge from the hospital wards." Their 1918 report added utilization of "all the sanitaria, convalescent homes, vacation funds, employment agencies and charitable agencies that may . . . help the patient or his family to pay for the medicine, apparatus, or vacation that may assure recovery."

In 1914 the trustees appointed Miss Ida Cannon Chief of Hospital Social Service. The service developed rapidly and in 1919 was made a department of the hospital. In 1930 the service was extended to the McLean Hospital (a psychiatric inpatient facility in suburban Belmont) and to the newly opened Baker Memorial division of the M.G.H. This established the fact that social service is needed at all economic levels.

By 1935 Dr. Washburn could write, "No hospital in the U.S. of any size worthy of the name is without such a department, and in many other countries the example has been followed."[26]

Expensive? Yes, very. The departmental expenses in 1918 were roughly $25,000, while in 1968 they exceeded $400,000.

The value of the contributions, however, cannot be priced. Today, the Department of Social Service is a vital example of the social conscience of the hospital, its determination to fulfill its primary function. Never has it been more important to have such a department. With its aid we have been able to reduce length of stay and improve the utilization of expensive technology, obtain the best extended-care facilities for our patients, and foster improvement in the development and function of such facilities.

The Baker Memorial Hospital and Fee Plan of 1930

In 1917 Phillips House had opened, providing for the first time completely private rooms for the well-to-do. But there remained a large segment of the population unable to afford private care and yet not qualified for admission to the general hospital and its wards.

[26] *Ibid.*, p. 467.

As Washburn had said in 1914, "This group in the community must often be ill in their homes, dependent upon physicians who cannot provide the necessary laboratory tests and scientific examinations which are readily available in the general hospital."[27]

In 1930 the Baker Memorial Hospital for patients of moderate means was opened. Patients were admitted if they fell within certain income limits; the average income of patients admitted during the first year of operation was $2,101.74. Hospital charges ranged from $4.50 per day in a four-bed room to $6.50 for a single room. The staff had agreed to a hospital-regulated set of fees with a maximum of $150 no matter how long the patient stayed or how complex the condition. Washburn wrote: "The Massachusetts General Hospital is blessed with a medical and surgical staff which is public spirited and desires to cooperate with the Hospital in any progressive movement for the good of the community. Of its own volition the staff has agreed to accept at the Baker Memorial a small regulated fee for its professional services."[28]

In its first year the average all-inclusive charge was $158.94; the average length of stay was thirteen days. Fifteen per cent of the patients needed special nursing care with an average additional charge of $121.40, demonstrating vividly how important and costly was special nursing care, even in 1930.

The experiment succeeded; the patient of moderate means was indeed protected from excessive hospital costs and professional fees. Here stands a second example of cooperative institutional effort to solve pressing social and economic problems of medicine—doctors, administration, and trustees working side by side to utilize the maximum potential of the hospital as a social instrument.

The Emergency Ward

Today one of the most useful measures of a hospital's ability and willingness to serve its community is the functioning of its emergency department: Are its facilities open twenty-four hours a day,

[27] *M.G.H. Annual Report, 1914*, pp. 61–62.

[28] Washburn, *The Massachusetts General Hospital*, pp. 249–250.

seven days a week? Does it accept alcoholic patients? Is its service predicated by need, or determined by the patient's ability to pay? In short, has it become the sanctuary for the fulfillment of human need in time of suffering, anxiety, distress, or disaster? If any of these questions are answered negatively, it has not optimally fulfilled what the community wants and needs today. Indeed, what it expects in the current turmoil of the medical-care system of our country is to be found in this department of the hospital.

Looking Ahead

Where does the hospital go from here? Is the emergency ward truly to remain a "sanctuary," or can we do better for our ever-growing population? I believe our urban hospitals are the logical institutions from which *actively* to extend our services—our people and our knowledge—to urban *and* suburban regions where need and demand are mounting rapidly. Through coordinated regional planning, more people will be served at a lower cost and much of our present system of medical care and preventive medicine will be improved.

Our teaching hospitals are called "health centers" today, when, in reality, they enjoy a limited and exclusive function as the citadels of acute, curative, scientific, and technical medicine. Medical educators speak of comprehensive medical care as including the preservation of health and the prevention as well as the cure of disease. Continuity of care and home care are stressed. The aims of such "comprehensive" care are laudable, but they are rarely achieved, except for the "cure of disease" part. As the successes of medical science and medical technology pile up, the subdivision of medical labor increases, with its attendant technical competence, discontinuity of care, manpower shortages, and high cost. These considerations prevent the giving of comprehensive care and the development of the true "health center"—a focal point for community health care. Obviously, our educational system and the "learning field" in medicine must be considered deficient if they evade the study of social and economic dis-ease manifested, respectively, by the expanding numbers of what we call the "mentally ill" and the increasing difficulty in financing the care of the chronically ill as they steadily enlarge our aged population. Similarly, the availability and utilization of health services remain uneven; those most in need—the impoverished, our children, and the aged—find themselves least able to satisfy their needs.

All roads in the community lead to the "health centers" which find themselves restricted to the treatment of established somatic disease by teams of specialists. There is no public health or preventive medicine discipline available. Many hospitals have no social service and, at best, only poorly developed outpatient ambulatory clinics. There is no honest attempt to provide continuity of care or extension of services to the community and into the home. There is little coordination or communication with the other caring institutions of the community—nursing homes, homemaker services, rehabilitation services, visiting nurse associations, churches, schools, courts of law, urban renewal organizations—and the care of the mentally ill has long since been segregated and resides in distant asylums, public and private. The hospital has emerged in the eyes of the profession as the "medical center" only because of its central position in the successful treatment of somatic crises.

The health of a community must inevitably include considerations of its economic, educational, recreational, and general social condition. Somatic and psychic disease is most prevalent in urban, impoverished communities where, hand in hand, one finds the poorest living conditions, highest unemployment rates, lowest educational facilities and attainment, and the greatest civil unrest. Inevitably, medicine must concern itself with the larger field of social welfare and develop a holistic concept of a community's health, if it is to prevent disease, maintain health, and thereby enhance the quality of life, to say nothing of the national welfare. Such a concept will allow medicine to take its rightful place in the larger field of social welfare and will considerably enhance the learning experience of *all* health personnel. Simultaneously, it will allow study and experimentation with the better use of scarce health personnel and the more rational use of health services by the community. The cost of such services, although increased when provided initially to such deprived communities, should be more than justified through the economic advantages of preventing disease, or of rehabilitating those with disease, to say nothing of the better use of lower-cost facilities (than hospitals) where appropriate. I believe the urban hospitals (largely teaching hospitals) must take the lead in such developments, for they alone have the resources of sufficient concentration to do the job.

The M.G.H. has developed such a holistic plan in conjunction with all the organizations concerned with the health of a community —whether urban renewal, political education, welfare, religion, public health and visiting nurse services, or others. It is the over-all aim of this program to develop a health service system which will represent all the resources required to cultivate high-level physical and psychologic health and to prevent, detect, and treat disease and disability, as needed to maintain optimal health throughout life.

As of this writing, we have joined with the Department of Health and Hospitals of the City of Boston to develop the M.G.H.–Bunker Hill Health Center in Charlestown (a subdivision of Boston). The Health Center has been in operation for several months. Its initial operations have been described in the *M.G.H. News* of February 1969 as follows:

> A community that never before had specialists such as internists or pediatricians working in it, Charlestown is beginning to experience the luxury of comprehensive medical care in its most modern form.
>
> The M.G.H. center took its first halting step in September by assuming from the city of Boston the health services of Charlestown's seven public schools. A grant from the Children's Bureau of the Department of Health, Education and Welfare made that beginning possible.
>
> On January 1, the center added the three parochial schools. Now the red-brick building serves a total of 4,500 children.
>
> January 1 also saw the center take over the personal health care services previously carried out in Charlestown by the Boston Department of Health and Hospitals.
>
> It opened its doors to all ages and income groups at that time, bringing the entire family into the health picture. . . . Until last fall, Charles-

town was like any one of hundreds of American communities gripped by a medical manpower shortage. The shortage translated itself to inadequate and fragmented care.

In a spot check last May of 205 Charlestown children pre-registered for kindergarten and the first grade:

1) Only 68 per cent had the basic immunization series against diphtheria, whooping cough and tetanus.
2) Only 42 per cent had a booster.
3) Only 61 per cent were fully immunized against polio.
4) Only 41 per cent had measles shots.

"We now have both the availability and accessibility of care which can change statistics like these," said Dr. John P. Connelly, Executive Director of the center.

Few of the changes being made in Charlestown are strikingly new. For the first time, however, the services are being provided in a coordinated way.

"In school health," Dr. Connelly said, "we are providing a central service for all facets of care instead of the isolated and fragmented manner of yesterday. In one sitting, we test hearing, vision, blood, urine, blood pressure, and vital signs, take growth measurements, get a complete medical history and give a physical examination. When needed, we are backed up by the specialty care available at the M.G.H. . . . Thus we provide a comprehensive overview of the health of the children."

One example of a new service is the throat culture. The state has offered throat-culturing facilities for many years. Until the establishment of the M.G.H.–Bunker Hill Health Center, however, there was no system designed to reach the Charlestown patients at highest risk—the children.

Now throat cultures are becoming a routine part of the center's school health program. They are sent to state laboratories for examination. If positive, calls are made to the center, which then arranges for appropriate treatment and follow-up.

"We are uncovering a lot of strep infections in the throat," Dr. Connelly said. By treating the strep throats, the center can prevent rheumatic fever and the serious kidney ailment, nephritis. . . .

The same type of comprehensive medical care is beginning to be offered to Charlestown adults. The M.G.H. center, for example, has taken over the diabetes and tuberculosis programs and public health nursing services. . . .

Besides the major collaboration of the Boston Department of Health and Hospitals, the M.G.H. is working closely with several other organizations to provide high quality, personalized health, social and educational services to its patients.[29]

Several important developments should be noted:

(1) The effort represents a public-private coordinated endeavor.

(2) Local community physicians have not been displaced and are, in fact, active participants of importance of the first order.

(3) Acute curative services, preventive as well as diagnostic, are offered.

(4) A multidisciplinary approach, regionally planned, is in operation.

(5) The entire endeavor is being carefully and extensively researched from the standpoint of costs and benefits, the national development of comprehensive and preventive services, and the better use of scarce manpower.

(6) When the program is well established, teaching will become an active part for *all* students of relevant disciplines—medicine, nursing, social sciences, and so on.

(7) The services must be developed for acceptance by *all* social and economic classes and not just the impoverished white community of Charlestown.

(8) The M.G.H. will work toward complete responsibility for the ongoing operations of the center—although the federal grant was absolutely necessary to initiate the project. The multiplicity of overlapping federal programs must be simplified in order to encourage such developments.

In summary, the hospital has evolved from a house of despair for the sick poor to the modern house of hope for all social and economic classes. It is now the major urban social institution which has the resources and capacity to extend itself actively out into the community. In planned coordination with all individuals and organ-

[29] M. Bander, "Center Is Improving Care in Charlestown," *M.G.H. News* 28 (February 1969): 1.

izations concerned with community health, the hospital can reach more people with its diagnostic and preventive services. It can research and improve the present system of medical care and ultimately contain costs through the earlier detection of disease, the maintenance of health, the prevention of illness, and the more efficient use of scarce manpower and costly technology.

Acknowledgment: Some of the material for this paper has previously been published in J. H. Knowles, "The Social Conscience and the Primary Function of the Hospital Viewed in Historical Perspective," *The Pharos of Alpha Omega Alpha* 26 (July 1963): 67.

The Coming Revolution in Medicine: A New Plan for Ambulatory Medical Care

DAVID D. RUTSTEIN, M.D.

Ridley Watts Professor of Preventive Medicine and Head of the Department Harvard University Medical School

IF ANYONE IS SICK ENOUGH to need a doctor, but not so ill as to be flat in bed in a hospital, the chances are that he will not get the full benefits of modern medical care. In the United States, ambulatory medicine—the care of the patient "on the hoof"—tends to be catch as catch can, particularly if he has an acute medical or surgical emergency, if he needs preventive services, or if he is suffering from a minor illness or the early stages of a serious disease. In sharp contrast, in many of our hospitals, particularly those affiliated with medical schools, the care of the patient may be the best in the world.

Let us examine each of these varieties of unsatisfactory ambulatory care. Emergency care may be unnecessarily delayed and is often inadequate. Communication between the emergency case and the treatment center is casual, transportation may be hit or miss, and each medical and surgical emergency station operates in its own self-centered way. Haphazard distribution and operation of emergency facilities may result in the loss of precious time as the patient is shipped from hospital to hospital in search of the necessary specialized care. Witness the delay in the treatment of the late Senator Robert F. Kennedy in Los Angeles when, with a bullet in his brain, he was rushed to a hospital that was unable to care for him. He had then to be transferred to another hospital equipped and staffed to cope with brain injuries. As events proved, the loss of time in his treatment probably made no difference in the outcome, but in some cases unnecessary delay and disorganization may make the difference between life and death.

When the patient needs preventive care or ambulatory treatment for a minor complaint, which may be the early stage of a major illness, the hospital may be inadequately supported by modern technology and lack easy access to needed specialists' services. During the day a private patient will probably be treated in a doctor's office, relatively isolated from the complex panoply of technological facilities and the roster of specialists needed for complete medical care. Even if the physician's office is in a "group practice unit," the patient may not receive complete ambulatory care. Indeed, the phrase "group practice" may be misleading. Group practice units vary all the way from an office in which two physicians share the services of a secretary or a small laboratory, to well-organized care centers. But very few freestanding group practice units have available for their ambulatory patients the complete roster of specialists, paramedical personnel, and technological resources that are now the hallmark of modern scientific inpatient care.

If the patient cannot afford a private physician, he will be forced during the day to seek ambulatory care in the outpatient department of a hospital. Outpatient departments tend to be run in a relatively mechanical and impersonal fashion, often with interminable delays in unattractive surroundings. Among the worst examples are the outpatient prenatal-care clinics in New York City. According to the New York City Maternity Center Association, just under half (47 per cent) of the women delivered in municipal hospitals and slightly more than one third (34.5 per cent) of those delivered on the wards of voluntary hospitals in 1961 had not had the benefit of a single visit to a physician prior to delivery. The association ascribes the unwillingness of pregnant women to seek prenatal care to inadequate facilities and lack of system, including long waits under circumstances where toilet facilities may be completely lacking, and where no provisions exist for the care of the patients' other children.

The result of such inadequacy is an infant mortality rate twice as high as that of babies born to mothers with adequate prenatal care. Of course, there is a wide range of quality in the outpatient facilities of our many hospitals, and a few do provide good ambulatory care. But, for the country as a whole, the flat statement may be made that our hospital outpatient departments do not provide modern personal scientific medical care.

At night, ambulatory medical care may be even worse, for private and clinic patients alike. Private medical care is now almost completely unavailable at night. There is only one resource to which to turn—the emergency service of the local hospital, if any. Treatment there tends to be episodic, with little continuity of care. Physician and patient are usually complete strangers to each other and (probably) unlikely to see each other again.

Medical Care for the Poor

The glaring deficiencies in ambulatory medical care in the United States have been sharply focused by recent attempts to extend such care to disadvantaged populations. Although federal financing has been essential, the nature of medical care in poverty areas has been shaped mostly by local conditions—accessibility to a hospital and to a medical school, availability of empty buildings in the area, the interest and prejudices of physicians, local officials, and the residents of the area, and the marshaling of financial resources.

No single national pattern of medical care in disadvantaged areas has emerged. In general, three separate patterns have evolved. A few units have gotten underway, directed by medical school faculties or hospital research units (e.g., the Columbia Point Program in Boston and the Morrisania Program in the Bronx). They provide high-quality medical care, but their cost and elaborate professional staffing requirements make them nonreproducible as a general pattern for the entire country. Indeed, some academic experimental units are having increasing difficulty in recruiting for their own programs an adequate number of physicians and other professional staff. They may not be able to continue as originally planned.

At the other extreme, representatives of disadvantaged populations and their friends, sometimes aided by the local medical school, usually under inspired and devoted local leadership (e.g., Watts), have designed and built treatment centers from scratch. Ambulatory medical care is provided where for all practical purposes none previously existed. But such centers tend to be relatively isolated from technological resources and specialists' services and have great difficulty in physician recruitment. Indeed, after the initial flurry of excitement has died down, health departments and other agencies working with local community groups have over the years found it almost impossible to recruit enough competent physicians to provide medical care in centers remote from hospitals. Isolation from professional contacts and hospital resources, inadequate financial compensation, and the waste of professional time in transportation in our heavily trafficked cities or in driving long distances out in the country are probably responsible for the lack of success of this kind of ambulatory medical care.

Ambulatory care has also been provided in disadvantaged areas by the extension of existing outpatient hospital services. These efforts have been relatively unsuccessful because of their intrinsic limitations, their functional separation from the inpatient-care resources of the hospital, and the impersonal isolation of the clinic from the patient population served in the community.

And yet all these efforts must be applauded, because services are provided in areas where none previously existed. Medical-care programs for the poor have certainly satisfied many unmet needs. From a short-range point of view, such efforts are and have been useful and should be supported. The best must not become the enemy of the good. But we must also take the long view. We must eventually develop a system of ambulatory services that at one and the same time fosters personal care and brings all of the benefits of modern scientific medicine to all of our citizens.

How then can we design and test an ambulatory medical-care program that will favor a personal physician-patient relationship, implement modern scientific knowledge, incorporate relevant advances in modern technology, supply essential specialist services, and apply existing and potential social resources for the benefit of all patients?

Let us begin by making sure, in the process of introducing a new system of ambulatory care, that no patient is harmed. Although planning the total program should begin immediately, the emergency medical service has first priority, in order to assure effective treatment of surgical and medical emergency cases. Since emergency care tends to be chaotic, we must first concentrate on developing and testing an effective emergency-care program. This process should not interfere with total program planning or with the implementation of feasible parts of it. If the emergency medical program is successful, it will save lives threatened in surgical and medical emergencies and make the total program more acceptable. Moreover, with the assurance of effective treatment for such emergencies, we will be able to take a more thoughtful and thoroughgoing approach to the design and testing of an efficient ambulatory medical-care program in a complete medical-care system.

Emergency Medical Service

The armed forces have had the greatest experience in caring for acute emergencies. It has often been said that a soldier in Vietnam receives far more effective emergency care than an injured civilian on a modern American superhighway. Military experience has demonstrated the need for three major interrelated constituents, all of which are lacking in most civilian emergency medical services. The essentials are (1) an areawide communications system that interrelates with (2) a transportation system geared to meet geographic and strategic needs, and (3) a series of interrelated emergency-care centers designed to treat specifically defined medical and surgical problems. Such programs have been validated in Vietnam to a point where there is no longer any need for the services of a battalion surgeon in the front lines. With efficient communication and transportation and a medical corpsman to provide first aid, the military patient is cared for in a hospital behind the lines by a physician who has at hand the benefits of technological, medical, paramedical, and specialist support—that is, all the essential constituents of modern medical care.

The translation of the principles learned in military emergency programs to the civilian scene should not be overly difficult. And yet the relative lack of experience with civilian systems of emergency care demand that initial efforts be established as pilot experiments. Development of a model will demand the collaborative efforts of communications and transportation engineers, systems analysts, operations research experts, physicians, public health and hospital administrators, paramedical personnel, and biostatisticians. Most important, practical implementation will require close working relationships with a committee consisting of representatives of the community.

Urban and rural emergency-care systems are essentially the same in principle. Both are based on the triad of efficient communications and transportation, and specifically designed emergency-care stations. Minor modifications of details may be needed to meet local needs.

The emergency medical program will be coordinated by an area-wide network flowing into a communications center. The communications network must include every telephone in the local system (including pay telephones where emergency calls may be made without the use of a coin, by dialing a special number), communications posts in police cars, ambulances, fire apparatus, taxis, and common carriers. Emergency phones must be placed along the highways, particularly at points where accidents are frequent. Highway mileposts (similar to those in European countries, where every tenth of a kilometer is marked), will be needed for precise location of accident sites. A signaling system for passing motorists will have to be created. A public education program on personal injury and accident reporting will have to be instituted, conducted, and tested. Stress must be placed on the threat to the system and the danger to individuals in the community if the network becomes clogged by false alarms.

The communications center must be manned by personnel competent to evaluate each case, perform triage,[1] refer the patient to the appropriate emergency station, and then select and dispatch the most

[1] This term, coming into civilian use, is an adaptation of the military term that denotes the process by which injured soldiers are sorted out on the battlefield for transfer to the most appropriate medical-care facility.

appropriate emergency transportation vehicle—whether ambulance, taxi, personal automobile, police car, helicopter, airplane, or common carrier.

In studies performed in the Family Health Program of the Massachusetts General Hospital in the 1950's, it was demonstrated that a specially trained public health nurse with access to a physician's advice by telephone can evaluate medical and surgical problems and perform effective triage. Studies will determine whether a nurse can also serve effectively in an emergency-care system, and work in collaboration with a transportation expert.

The transportation expert will have complete control over all vehicles used in the transportation of emergency cases. Every vehicle transporting critically ill patients must be manned by personnel trained to perform first aid and resuscitation, to splint fractures, and to carry injured and seriously ill patients. The transportation expert must be capable of understanding the nature of medical and surgical emergencies and the reasons for transportation to a particular emergency station.

Fortunately, there exists a large untapped pool of trained personnel to do this job. Military corpsmen, well trained in emergency care, are constantly being discharged back to their communities, where there are few if any opportunities to use their special skills and to earn adequate compensation therefor. Indeed, most military corpsmen upon discharge from the armed services take other kinds of jobs because the only medical job opening in most communities is that of hospital orderly. Rarely, corpsmen may be employed as "physician's assistants" or in other paramedical positions in academically oriented experiments in medical care. The discharged medical corpsmen have exactly the training and skills needed to provide medical care on emergency vehicles. The emergency medical-care program badly needs their services and skills. With the scarcity of medical personnel, we can ill afford to waste this valuable resource.

The number of emergency treatment stations should be determined by the needs of the community. There need not be an emergency treatment center in every hospital. Indeed, because of the requirement for twenty-four hour coverage, emergency stations can be located only in hospitals having a resident staff. But every hospital must be tied in to the emergency medical service if only to guide to proper care the cases coming to its attention.

Depending upon hospital resources, availability of specialized physicians and other personnel, laboratory facilities, and equipment, some stations may treat all emergencies; others may treat only medical or surgical cases; while still others may have the professional, technological, and technical personnel to provide such highly specialized care as that demanded by cardiac emergencies or head injuries.

A well-functioning emergency medical service would meet the needs of physicians and the public. All would learn of the benefits of a systematic attack on an important medical-care problem. Most physicians are not interested in providing twenty-four hour a day emergency service for which they are poorly compensated. Physicians would appreciate the opportunity to refer their emergency cases if they had the assurance that their patients would be well treated. The physician would also become aware that the introduction of a system per se need not threaten his independence nor the physician-patient relationship. The public would be reassured that their emergency needs would be systematically cared for with immediate access to necessary personnel, equipment, and other resources.

We can no longer be satisfied with the hodgepodge of emergency treatment centers that willy-nilly provide or refuse care to those who knock at their doors. We cannot continue to refer patients to "the nearest hospital" (as is provided by police regulations in some of our larger cities) without regard to the nature of the emergency or to the resources available for treatment. Moreover, our limited health budgets cannot tolerate the wasteful duplication of emergency stations in our haphazard lack of system. When we face up to all these facts, we realize that there is no choice but to create a central emergency authority in each population center to plan, introduce, integrate, and supervise all aspects of the system to the end that each emergency case receives at the earliest possible moment exactly the treatment needed.

The Total Program

A total ambulatory medical-care program incorporating the emergency-care system cannot be started everywhere at once and might best be tested in urban poverty areas. The needs there are greatest and the benefits most easily evaluated. The decision to begin in a poverty area does not in any way imply that disadvantaged groups should have a different kind of medical care than the rest of the population. Indeed, the opposite is the case. If the expectations for a carefully planned systematic ambulatory program are borne out, there should be a general demand for its extension to other areas, to do away with such frequent complaints as "We don't have a doctor in our town"; "You can't ever get to see a doctor when you need one"; "The doctor is booked for weeks ahead"; "You wait all day in the outpatient department and finally you see a different doctor every time." The proposed model program should be applicable not only to other urban areas but with some modification in transportation facilities to rural areas as well.

Finally, the introduction of a new system, to replace the present unplanned "cottage industry" of ambulatory medical care, demands carefully controlled evaluation as a guide for the future. It is impossible to begin new, complete, ambulatory-care systems in all urban disadvantaged areas in large cities at the same time. Advantage should be taken of this limitation to make the control observations essential to a precise evaluation of the new system. If two similar adjacent areas can be selected and one of them chosen randomly as a site of the new program, control measurements may be made in the other, where one of the usual varieties of poverty-area programs (that is, the creation of an area-centered treatment center) would be put in operation.

Let us define the essentials of an ambulatory medical-care system, go through the stages of its organization, and demonstrate how a member of the community would be cared for and benefited.

The essentials of an effective ambulatory medical-care program would include (1) an educational program to institute and maintain a close working relationship between the patients and the medical-care staff; (2) a reception and triage center conveniently located in the geographic area served by the program; (3) a health department alerting system to identify the preventive and therapeutic needs of individual residents; (4) a treatment center adjacent to the local hospital and functionally interrelated with its technological resources and specialist services; (5) a communications system to guarantee the most efficient interrelationship of all facilities for the care of the individual patient; (6) a special transportation system linking the home of the patient with all units where prevention or treatment may be given; (7) a center for the temporary care of children of mothers needing medical treatment; and (8) an affiliation of the ambulatory-care program through the local hospital with the regional medical-care system.

The Educational Program. The residents of the community must have a clear understanding of the objectives of the program. They must know that an unusual variety of ambulatory care is being provided for them which should be better than the mere availability of a physician. They must learn why a physician alone cannot practice modern scientific medicine and why he needs systematic support from professional and technological personnel as well as the use of modern medical machinery. They must agree that the time of the physician has to be reserved for those tasks only he can perform. They must accept services from specially trained paramedical personnel that formerly were provided by a physician. Finally, they must collaborate in an educational program that will keep them informed so that they may derive maximum benefits from the program. Toward these ends, the planning committee of the program must include among its membership many of the leaders of the community.

The Reception Center. The focal point of contact between the residents of the community and the ambulatory-care system is the reception center, which has to be conveniently located in the heart of the area and should preferably be housed in the local urban services center. The staff of the reception center would consist of specially trained public health nurses, paramedical assistants (perhaps military corpsmen), and secretarial and clerical aides. The regional staff would use the reception center as their point of departure for home visits, as a first-aid station, and as a triage center for residents of the area seeking medical care.

Community liaison through the reception center would be greatly assisted by a well-organized health department alerting system. The local health department, working with the staff of the reception center, would collect current data on events having health and medical significance in the lives of community residents (as, for example, marriages, births, accidents, hospital admission), and significant laboratory reports, such as positive pregnancy, infectious disease, and biopsy tests. It would also keep a registry of the newborn and of the dates when preventive services (e.g., immunizations and nutritional supervision) were needed.

When alerted by one of these events, the public health nurse would make a home visit or arrange an appointment for a needed preventive or therapeutic service. Services to a community member by the public health nurse in time of need should aid in cementing personal relationships with the reception center staff and in building the confidence of the community in the ambulatory medical-care program.

Confidence is essential to community acceptance of new patterns of medical care. American patients able to afford a physician and needing medical care are accustomed to working with him alone, as if he were able to provide all aspects of care by himself. In this ambulatory program, the first contact would be made by a specially trained nurse and the patient would be referred to a physician when necessary. The residents of the community must be made aware that they will receive better medical care if their physician is supported by nurses and other paramedical personnel and buttressed by modern technological resources.

How would the nurse decide on referral to medical care? The nurse faced with a patient seeking help must make one of three decisions: (1) the patient is well and does not need the physician's care; (2) the patient is sick enough to need treatment immediately (or by appointment on the following day); or (3) further consultation is necessary. When the patient's complaint is minor, as, for example, a cut finger, immediate first aid should suffice and the "well" patient would be sent home, reassured, with instructions to return should an unusual complication supervene. At the other extreme, the sick patient would be transferred to the hospital immediately, or to the ambulatory treatment center on the same or on the following day, depending on how sick he was.

Studies on nurse triage in the Massachusetts General Hospital Home Care Program revealed that in the third case there were usually two reasons why the nurse herself could not make a decision as to the immediate need for a physician's care: the nurse's medical knowledge might not be adequate, or the disease might not yet have evolved to a point where even the most competent physician could make a diagnosis. In either event, consultation with a physician at another telephone on the same extension would yield an immediate decision as to the need for a physician's care, or for the institution of follow-up of the patient by the nurse. In the latter instance, follow-up would be continued until a decision could be made as to whether the patient merely needed reassurance or whether referral to a physician for appropriate medical care was necessary.

It is to be noted that the reception center does not have a physician on its staff. A physician could not practice modern medicine in the reception center without extensive and wasteful duplication of technological facilities and personnel already available in the nearest hospital. With efficient communications and with transportation systems available to transfer patients to physicians appropriately located to provide good care, there is no more need for a physician in the reception center, than for the battalion surgeon in Vietnam. He can be replaced by a public health nurse and the civilian equivalent of a medical corpsman. The physician's services can then be reserved for those medical procedures demanding his education, experience, knowledge, and skill.

The Treatment Center. Most ambulatory medical care will be provided by a physician in the treatment center located adjacent to the hospital, with immediate access to all of its resources.[2] The treatment center should have all the attributes not traditionally associated

[2] There may, of course, be other specialized ambulatory-care facilities, such as a mental health center, that must be functionally interrelated.

with outpatient hospital facilities. If possible, the building should be freestanding and not in the center of the maze of inpatient services, for such a maze is associated in the mind of the layman with the treatment of serious illness. And yet, there must be functional interrelationships with all laboratory, x-ray, and other technological facilities, with the record room, with the roster of specialists, and with the inpatient services when hospital admission is indicated. One might hope that the treatment center would be clean and attractive, with comfortable waiting rooms, adequate toilet facilities, and parking space for vehicles, including baby carriages. The appointment system should be efficient and geared to the employment schedules of the male patients and the family demands of the female patients. Triage service would be available for patients living in the neighborhood of the treatment center. In a word, the treatment center would be a place where the patient would receive kind, considerate, and scientific medical care in attractive surroundings.

Medical responsibility for the care of patients in the treatment center should be given to those physicians who can grace the solid framework of medical science with the kindly art of patient care. Under their supervision, much of the actual care, particularly in urban areas, would be provided by interns and residents. Exposing physicians-in-training to such ambulatory care would bring balance into that distorted scheme of postgraduate medical education which now focuses almost entirely on the diagnosis of complicated illness, the use of miracle drugs, and the mechanical relief of major difficulties by heroic surgery. Continuity of care will present a difficult problem, as physicians-in-training rotate and then leave to practice elsewhere. A permanent staff of supervisory physicians will have to bridge the gap.

The Group Practice Unit. The physicians on the hospital staff would be served best if their group practice offices were located in a building adjacent to the hospital. In such a location, their time could be devoted to professional tasks and not wasted in moving from place to place. Close at hand the physician would have available for his ambulatory patients the panoply of technological resources established for inpatient care. Moreover, if the ambulatory-care center were close to the group practice unit, specialist referral would be facilitated. A patient referred from the treatment center would be cared for in the office of a specialist in the unit. Specialists would then practice with a maximum of efficiency, since they could treat all their ambulatory patients in the same office.

Communications and Transportation Systems. The ambulatory program must have a communications system of its own, tying together in a communications center all the service units and the transportation system. When the total program is under way, the communications center of the emergency system would be interrelated.

Effective transportation for the users of the ambulatory-care system is a *sine qua non*. Residents in disadvantaged areas do not have easily available the kind of transportation that is needed for adequate medical care. Common carriers are often relatively inaccessible in disadvantaged areas, particularly at night. Furthermore, taxi services are hit or miss in low-income neighborhoods and they are too expensive for the average resident. A special transportation system is needed. It would operate between the home, reception center, ambulatory treatment center, hospital, and other referral facilities, as well as all units of the regional system. The transportation provided should be that demanded by the state of the patient's health. The vehicle might be a bus, private car, ambulance, or, in an emergency, a vehicle to provide the most rapid transportation to the appropriate emergency station. It goes without saying that the transportation system must also be fitted into the appointment system of all treatment units.

The system should not be designed solely for the transportation of extremely ill patients. It should be attractive enough to induce patients to seek preventive services, such as immunization or prenatal care, or to participate in a screening program for the early stages of serious illness. The transportation system must not act as a hindrance. On the contrary, it must be so efficient and attractive that patients will gladly use it in the early stages of illness to obtain effective care. Indeed, a transportation system focusing on preventive services should prove to be a good investment. The returns would include better health for the population and financial savings from the prevention of unnecessary hospital admissions.

Temporary Child-Care Center. The temporary child-care center or centers must be located close to the transportation system so that a mother requiring preventive or therapeutic treatment may be relieved of her children for the period of time needed for her medical care. The child-care center should be so operated that mothers will seek medical assistance, confident that their children will be well cared for in their absence.

A Regional System. Finally, if the local hospital with which the ambulatory center is affiliated were part of a regional system, the picture would be complete. For example, if the ambulatory system were adjacent to a community hospital and the patient needed super-specialists' care such as may be demanded by a difficult diagnosis or complicated (e.g., open-heart) surgery, the services could be brought to him, or, when necessary, he could be referred to the appropriate specialist in another hospital in the regional system.

Relating the proposed ambulatory program to the regional system has another advantage. It would not be necessary that there be a physician resident in every small community. The program would thus do away with the almost endless but pointless discussion on the place of residence of the practicing physician and focus instead on the availability of care to meet the preventive and therapeutic needs of the residents of the area. Thus, even in the absence of a physician resident in the community, good ambulatory care can be provided in both urban and rural areas if the communications and transportation systems interrelate the ambulatory medical-care program with local and regional resources.

The introduction of this new system of ambulatory care would also do away with some wasteful practices and should make medical care less expensive. In a word, it is time that medical care caught up with the industrial revolution and benefited from its greater efficiency. The "cottage industry" must come of age. There are many examples. The office of the individual practicing physician is improvident of capital investment and enhances operating costs. Some office space and the almost endlessly duplicated medical equipment, such as electrocardiographs and fluoroscopes, lie fallow many hours of the day. The patient's fee or insurance payment must of course cover these needless costs.

We may note another example. Insurance contracts (e.g., Blue Cross) pay for expensive laboratory services, such as gastrointestinal x-ray, only for patients in the hospital. Patients may often needlessly be put to bed for care that could be provided more cheaply, more efficiently, and more conveniently on an ambulatory basis. The waste does not end there. Unnecessary hospital admissions force the community to increase the size of its hospitals and maintain far more beds than are actually needed to provide good medical care for the residents of the community. The cost of superfluous hospital beds becomes all the more alarming as the cost of medical care continues to rise—far more rapidly than any other item in the Consumer Price Index—and, of all items of medical care, inpatient hospital care is rising most sharply.

More important, there are many potential medical benefits from the new ambulatory-care system: a more effective handling of emergency cases with the saving of lives; earlier treatment of many cases of serious illness; saving of the physician's time for those tasks that demand his unique capabilities; and more effective deployment of medical equipment and personnel for earlier and better diagnosis and treatment. We will all benefit by a decrease in disease and disability and in postponement of untimely death.

A Clinical Investigator Looks at Modern Education: The Discovery of the Medical Student as a Responsible Colleague

THOMAS HALE HAM, M.D.

Hanna Payne Professor of Medicine and Director of Research in Medical Education School of Medicine, Case Western Reserve University

Francis W. Peabody, founder of the Thorndike Memorial Laboratory at the Boston City Hospital, was one of the great clinicians, clinical investigators, and teachers of his time. His much admired essay entitled "The Care of the Patient" furnishes his approach to the patient.[1] The last sentence gives the key: "One of the essential qualities of the clinician is interest in humanity, for the secret of the care of the patient is in caring for the patient." In this presentation I shall look at medical education by the use of many of the methods described by Peabody, namely, those appropriate to the clinical investigator. By his methods we shall rediscover the needs of the student, the patient, the faculty, and also our administrative colleagues.

What methods of the clinical investigator lend themselves to this approach? First, he is trained to observe the manifestations of illness, in order to accomplish several objectives. He tries to clarify the problems of the patient and then to seek appropriate measure-

[1] Francis W. Peabody, "The Care of the Patient," *J.A.M.A.* 88 (March 19, 1927): 877–882.

ments of the symptoms, the signs, and the laboratory manifestations of illness. Ultimately, he tries to help the patient by procedures based on the clinical investigation itself. Not all illness can be expected to respond to this approach. However, the investigator constantly returns to the patient who must have help. The investigator is problem oriented and seeks the solution to the key problems, including participation from many colleagues in other fields, because the need is so great. The very statement of critical need leads to the development of new methods for measurement, for understanding, and, ultimately, for change in the care of the patient.

In the field of medical education it is quite apparent that we are dealing with many unknowns and that the needs are great, as they are in many branches of medicine. Often we are forced to approach education descriptively because our measurements are not yet adequate. Probably in the science of education we are still at about the year 1850 in comparison to the medical sciences, and we have not yet had a Pasteur to give us the understanding of yeast and microorganisms, nor a Koch to provide the postulates underlying causation of disease by organisms, nor a Lister to apply these to surgery.

In this presentation I intend to follow the history of medical education in the United States, beginning in 1634 and coming rapidly to the student in the Class of 1972. By this quick trip I should be able, as an investigator, to observe the true needs of the student during various periods of education in this country and then to define the role of the medical student in today's complex society. I shall show by example how the responsibility of the medical student can be increased by participation in learning with the patient, the faculty, and the administration. The next several decades are promising indeed, because the needs are so enormous that change is inevitable and will bring refreshment and challenge to each of us who joins in the process.

Preceptorial Period (1634–1765)

Anyone who wanted to study medicine in 1668—three centuries ago—would have found that there were no medical schools in the United States. In fact, there were none until late in 1765. For the study of medicine, then, in 1668, after completing his schooling, equivalent to contemporary high school, at about sixteen to eighteen years of age, the student would discover that the only alternative available was individual instruction under a physician-preceptor, usually in his own neighborhood, selected because of his reputation as a doctor. The student and his family, calling on the physician, would enter into a written agreement for a three-year period during which he would learn medicine, possibly as the only student.[2] His family would probably pay one hundred dollars a year for tuition to this preceptor, and he would live in the home of the physician. During the first year he would "read medicine" with the doctor, studying the doctor's books on anatomy, medicine, surgery, midwifery, materia medica, and botany. He would assist with the practice, prepare medication, and do chores in the office, the home, and the barn. He would hitch up the horse. In the second year he would "ride out" with the doctor, helping him on his calls, with surgery, and with the many aspects of his practice in the patient's home. He probably would do a dissection of a human body, sometimes legally, sometimes not. In the third year he would assist further and at the end of this time obtain a certificate of proficiency—if he were found competent to practice independently—that is, "to ride alone." He could not qualify until he reached the age of twenty-one, so he might continue as an apprentice for several more years. There were no internships. The excellence of preceptorship depended entirely on the physician himself, his training, his library, and his willingness to supervise his student. Originally preceptors came from England and the Continent where the schools of medicine were well established and others were being formed.

This was one-to-one instruction: the individual student was the prime object of the teacher. It was always possible, therefore, for the student to obtain answers quickly to the pedagogic questions that he has continued to ask down through the centuries. I shall return over and over again to these primary questions and to the attempts to

2 A. Flexner, *Medical Education in the United States and Canada*, Report of the Carnegie Foundation for the Advancement of Teaching, Bull. no. 4 (New York: Merrymount Press, 1910), reprinted 1950.

procure the answers to them, namely: (1) What is important? (2) How am I doing? (3) What is relevant to my professional work? (4) What is my individual status? Much of the preceptorial relation has been carried throughout three centuries and is still being used extensively. Students now have the privilege of clinical preceptors also; however, the pedagogic questions asked by the student in earlier days, easily answered then, are difficult to answer today. I shall trace quickly the treatment of the student as a learner through three centuries of medical education.

The Preceptor and the Medical School (1765–1893)

In 1800 there were only four medical schools, the University of Pennsylvania, Dartmouth Medical School, Harvard Medical School, and King's College (now Columbia University) Medical School. But between 1800 and 1900 more than 450 medical schools were founded, most of them proprietary, based on a few faculty members who lectured in a hall, and relied heavily on the preceptorship to provide much of the student's experience. The medical school in those days was considered a radical departure because the preceptorship was the major method for education and the newfangled centralized units for lectures and demonstrations were considered of doubtful benefit.

The student who wished to enter the Cleveland Medical College, which was the medical department of Western Reserve in 1852, could not have matriculated unless certified as having satisfactorily completed a full year of preceptorship with a recognized physician somewhere in the area of Ohio, New York, or Pennsylvania, and recommended by him for further education.[3] Instead of entering a program of sequential courses, he would have attended lectures for a period of eighteen weeks. There were only six professors, and for fifty dollars the student bought a ticket for each eighteen-week series of professors' lectures. He attended lectures most of the day, but he also saw demonstrations of all the known physiology of that time. After the eighteen weeks of didactic teaching, he returned to his

[3] J. T. Baughman, "A Study of Medical Education in the United States," *J. Med. Ed.* 33 (1958): 132.

preceptor for the rest of that year to assist with patients, but he was required once again to return to the school of medicine for a second round of lectures. They were precisely the same as the first, but it was considered wise to repeat the course. He did a dissection and wrote a thesis, and then progressed (or not), as the result of an examination, and returned once again to his preceptor. His final arbiters were a board of censors in his home community who authorized him to undertake the practice of medicine if passed by their evaluation. Thus, again he was eligible after three years to be a physician, if he was 21 years of age.

Accordingly, for a century, the role of the physician-preceptor was dominant and that of the medical school distinctly secondary. A faculty of six could readily take care of a class of at least seventy-five students in the school. As a consequence, the lecture and demonstration became an integral method in the organized educational endeavor they administered. Of course, many advanced students during this period took training in England or continental Europe under famous pathologists, physicians, obstetricians, and other specialists in Munich, Vienna, Leiden, London, and Edinburgh, so that though internships were not required and there was no residency program, at least a few physicians had an opportunity to perfect their skills, as much as the state of knowledge permitted.

It is worth noting that in some schools lectures alone were given and no particular skill was imparted by laboratory or other practical exercises. These schools made money from lecture fees and referral of patients.

The Student and the Departmentalized Curriculum (1893–1950)

Scientific and clinical advances, especially in the nineteenth century, were large indeed, forming a basis for the scientific medicine in the chemical and physical sciences, in anatomy, microbiology, physiology, and pathology, and in the clinical fields with the advent of asepsis and anesthesia for surgery. The number of scientific and medical publications in all fields reached sixty thousand per year and was overwhelming the faculty.

Medical education in the United States, which had consisted of only three years' schooling and which had therefore awarded a license in medicine at the age of twenty-one, was abruptly altered by The Johns Hopkins University School of Medicine in 1893, when it introduced its program requiring a total of eight years. Four years were specified for college and four for medicine, and the program was based on a graded curriculum and a departmentalized medical school. This was the first school of its kind in the United States and it set the example for the time to come. The preceptorship method of medical education was rendered obsolete as a single method of education because the Hopkins system made it impossible for any preceptor to impart the available knowledge.

The report by Abraham Flexner in 1910 extended the Hopkins system,[4] and a gradual movement occurred in the United States toward departmentalized schools with a graded curriculum and full-time faculty members. Between 1910 and 1925 proprietary schools disappeared. Excellence of research in the biologic sciences and in the clinical fields brought a wealth of knowledge and an increase in the number of journals published to more than five thousand annually. Subspecialties were developed rapidly, not only in medical sciences but also in the clinical fields, in which marked advances were being made. Medical schools had growing access to research funds and had developed large facilities for conducting research, so that medical colleges and hospitals became medical universities, quite sufficient unto themselves. Because of the emphasis on research in many institutions, it was difficult for faculty to participate in a comparable manner in teaching and patient care.

The patient in this century was "discovered" by the clinical investigator in medical centers. Clear benefits had been derived from the careful research devoted to the nature and cure of the patient's illness. Yet the medical center no longer had the same base in the community as did the individual preceptor of the earlier centuries, so that the relation of the patient to the teacher-preceptor and to the student had changed markedly. The patient was often observed only

[4] Flexner, *Medical Education in the United States and Canada.*

in an acute episode of illness in hospital or clinic, and little chance existed to know him as an individual in the community. The relationship of the individual doctor to the individual patient was likely to be of limited continuity only. It may be observed that a variety of legislative acts have been initiated recently that undoubtedly will affect greatly the medical schools and the student as an attempt is made to individualize the patient again and to distribute clinical care more rationally.

The problems facing the student had increased in the first fifty years of the twentieth century, in a departmentalized curriculum. It was becoming difficult for the student to get answers to the fundamental questions once so easily answered by his preceptor: namely, what is most important; how am I doing; what is relevant to my professional work; and what is my individual status? Instead, the student was overwhelmed, overstuffed, over-lectured to, and overcommitted by each department, which believed most sincerely that its area of responsibility was of primary importance. In some schools the educational environment had been affected adversely by such factors as authoritarianism, ridicule, fear of failure (used as a prod), extreme departmental competition for the student's attention, the use of examinations as a whip, and intense rivalry of students for grades. The patient was seen rarely in the first two years, and students may often have wondered why they had come to medical school, what the purpose of medicine was. An enormous emphasis was placed on detail in preclinical fields, and no attempt was made to provide for the application of this information to real patients. The educational environment was such that many students hated medical school, could hardly wait to finish it, and suffered great discomfiture from the teaching methods.

Thus, during a very short period, beginning with the founding of The Johns Hopkins Medical School and the development of new departments and a graded curriculum, excellence of research, excellence of specialized medicine, and great advances in preclinical and clinical fields became characteristic. The student, however, was often lost in this great morass of expanded and perfected knowledge, excellent as it may have been in the abstract. The pedagogic methods no longer gave him the kind of support that he had enjoyed from the preceptor. The patient had disappeared from the first two years of the student's educational experience, and when he did appear it was only as he presented a form of incidental illness, often very severe, for which there was no follow-up. Little personal contact with the patient occurred before or afterward.

REDISCOVERY OF THE STUDENT (1950–1969)

Beginning at mid-century the faculty of the School of Medicine at Western Reserve University rediscovered the *student* by analyzing his problems in a departmentalized curriculum.[5]

First, the faculty found that members of fourteen departments could serve as true representatives and as peers working together. This approach allowed the privilege of debate, the opportunity for change, and the development of great respect among specialties. Out of all the multiple variables in a complex school of medicine, it was possible to define the needs of the student and to arrange a curriculum as a sequence of subjects taught interdepartmentally.[6]

The Subject Committee, composed of teachers from a number of departments, has served for sixteen years to bring together multiple disciplines in the teaching of a particular subject. The faculty is continuing this approach, finding that it allows for change, rekindles enthusiasms, and encourages the development of fine teachers.

The departmental structure has not been threatened by this approach but has continued as a strong organizational feature of the school of medicine, even though the subject committees have carried on many of the teaching programs.[7] The processes that have evolved governmentally include the development of policy for the education of the student by the democratic means of faculty peers working together. Once the general policy has been approved, it is administered

[5] T. H. Ham, "Medical Education at Western Reserve University: Progress Report for Sixteen Years, 1946–1962," *New England J. Med.* 267 (1962): 868–916.

[6] T. H. Ham, "Research in Medical Education: Participation of Faculty and Students," *Ann. New York Acad. Sci.* 128 (2) (1965): 501–518.

[7] T. H. Ham, "The Approaches of the Faculty to Medical Education at Western Reserve University," *J. Med. Educ.* 34 (12) (1959): 1163–1174.

by an assistant dean. The coordinators and departments continue to be the home base for fourteen different groups of colleagues who participate in research, in teaching graduate and postgraduate students, and in caring for patients.

A realignment took place in which the school of medicine discovered that one of its major purposes was planning and administering a program for student participation in learning. This approach reverses the usual pyramidal concept of an organizational plan, so that the student is now placed on the top and other units provide the infrastructure. This leadership from the dean up through the faculty to the student may be the needed relation for solving student-university problems in the future. It still permits self-discipline for all participants, and it leads to colleagueship with the student, who is rapidly led to feel that it is his responsibility to learn on his own.

Treatment of the Student as a Responsible Colleague

From the outset of the revision of the program of medical education it was considered essential that the educational environment for the student be appropriate to the growth of a responsible member of the school of medicine. This was stated explicitly as policy and was followed carefully from the time initial plans were created in 1952.[8] I quote:

> It is essential that the MD-student be treated as a maturing individual, as a colleague and as a student in a graduate professional school who is given increasing responsibility for his own education, for a knowledge of medicine and for the care of patients. This requires a mature system for examination and grading of the student and encouragement of the student initiative and resourcefulness. For example, in each year the MD-student might be given time for elective studies or courses and for conduct of unassigned work on the initiative of the student in such activities as organization and digestion of information, reading and interpretation of literature, preparation of reports, study of problems or cases, and conduct of research.

8 "Objectives concerning Curriculum," Committee on Medical Education, Draft no. 11 (April 10, 1951). These are minutes submitted to the General Faculty.

Key concepts introduced in this quoted policy include treating the student as a *maturing individual* and *colleague*. This approach was seriously challenged by some faculty members, who feared the student might be misled or treated too gently, as a colleague. They forgot how vigorously the faculty treated one another as colleagues. Stress was placed on the idea of a student in a graduate professional school who is given increasing responsibility for his own education.

Since 1952, the environment of the student has remained one that places increasing responsibility upon him. Instruction is gradually being transformed to meet the needs of the individual student, to make learning more effective, to evaluate learning, and to experiment with major factors influencing learning. The faculty is gradually transforming didactic teaching to teaching by student participation. Knowing where a student is, knowing how he functions, how to enter his mind, and how to train him in clear thinking about multiple problems are central to this process.[9] In this transformation of instruction, four postulates have been derived that appear essential for effective learning by the student. It will be helpful to put these postulates to test in the years to come so that they may be better defined and better evaluated for their significance. There are many curricula in the world of contemporary medical instruction, and this variety indicates that no one system has been established as the best. Conversely, the processes suggested in the following four postulates may be primary to any curriculum, and to any student of any age.

Postulate 1. Caring about the student. It is proposed that the process of caring about the student will literally discover the student who has a career as an individual as the unit of education. With the individual student as the basis for planning, the professional needs can be fitted to his learning level. To do so requires knowing where the student is and where he is going. Measurement can include exploring how the student progresses from one step to another in

[9] L. W. Weed, *The Problem-Oriented Record as a Basic Tool. Medical Records, Medical Education and Patient Care* (Cleveland: The Press, Case Western Reserve University, 1969).

knowledge, his use of information, and his perception of the educational process, that is, his educational environment.

Postulate 2. Informing the student what is important. The student will demand from his faculty some estimate of what is considered important for him to learn. Without such estimates he is quite lost. The explicit definition of objectives and competencies expected of each student must therefore be undertaken. Measurement can include evaluation of the student's perception of the use of the objectives in learning.

Postulate 3. Guiding the student in learning. The faculty will guide the individual student as the student learns on his own. The faculty must therefore consciously plan the kinds of instruction that will help the student accomplish the objectives developed for him. Measurement can include the responses of the student to many kinds of instruction and their effectiveness.

Postulate 4. Helping the student find out how he is progressing. Unable to judge his own performance, the student feels unable to guide himself in his own studying, lacks confidence in his progress, and therefore loses the satisfaction of accomplishment in the learning process. The faculty should provide methods of self-evaluation for the student as he learns content and process. The faculty will evaluate performance based on the objectives of its instruction. Evaluation procedures within a school and among schools must be developed in order to test learning of content and process and to obtain information about different kinds of instruction. Measurement can include the actual participation and satisfaction of the student in self-evaluation and in learning from the process of that evaluation. The faculty will measure performance of the individual student compared to that of students in general. Different instructional materials and methods will also be evaluated.

Only a beginning has been made in carrying out the four postulates stated above, but many subject committees working together have developed their pedagogy to fit these approaches. It is immediately apparent, for example, that students recognize when the faculty is "*for* the student"—when the program has been designed for the true needs of the student rather than for the convenience of the faculty. It is apparent that when the student is expected to do a great deal for himself and is given the help he needs to permit him to do it, he responds creatively and emphatically. In spite of these idealistic approaches, however, the number of traditional lectures is still enormous and the need for pedagogic reform is still large.

Basically encouraging is a willingness on the part of faculty members to consider the important model for education that begins with the way the student is treated, where he stands in his learning process, and what should be done to plan his education. There is a willingness to give responsibility clearly to the student and to make that responsibility reasonable in kind and amount. Treatment of the student as a colleague has meant sharing the rationale of the educational program, that is, justifying the content and the educational approach. This has required an explicit analysis of the value and limitations of the program. It has meant expecting excellence of the student, who is joining the faculty in reaching out into the unknown. It has meant on all sides learning how to learn. More specifically, the objectives and competencies are being redefined by experts for the student so that he may understand exactly what is expected of him. That is, it has been necessary to define core knowledge, to take a problem-oriented approach, and to build the processes by which the student may extend his knowledge on his own. Once the student knows where he is in relation to learning objectives, he is in a position to proceed considerably with his own education, and the instructional method becomes a series of guidance systems in which the student participates. The student develops much of the initiative to choose his own form of instruction. A careful sequence would be recommended (primarily to save his time), and he would be offered also a variety of guidance aids—lectures, syllabi, texts, problems, unknowns and knowns, laboratory exercises, self-study units, and demonstrations.

The evaluation becomes a potential learning experience of great importance when it is conducted so that the student may know how he is progressing and how he can learn more. It is now evident that he will proceed on his own if this information is available. "Qualifying" becomes a final stage of responsibility in which the student demonstrates that he possesses the competencies outlined for him. The student-faculty interchange can be a continuing one in the interest of improving the above processes in learning.

Student Participation

Gradually, student participation has increased in the School of Medicine at Case Western Reserve University. It has been halting and timorous, because neither group involved could be confident of the appropriate contribution of each in coming together. But the policy is clear enough, as set forth in 1950 in a statement of the General Faculty, as follows:[10]

> It is believed that the program of medical education can be evolved in a continuing and experimental manner, with freedom of discussion, with opportunity to disagree and with opportunity for departments, faculty, and students to cooperate.
>
> Article x. *Student Participation.* It is understood that students will be invited to participate in a contributing manner to the Committee on Medical Education. Members of the Student Council, or other individual students, may be guests of the Committee at regular meetings or at specially arranged meetings. Students will be kept informed of the objectives of the Committee and its procedures to enlist their constructive cooperations in the planning and evaluation of the medical program.

It has been seventeen years since the setting was established for faculty-student interchange, and progress has been made slowly, but definitely. In the last three years real form has come to this cooperative endeavor, and it is now an accepted phenomenon as part of the ongoing program of the School of Medicine. Examples are given, as follows, in chronological order.

Reports of Students to the Coordinators. From the beginning of the new alignment of subject committees, the three coordinators, one for the first year (Phase I), one for the second and third years

[10] *Organization and Rules of Procedure for the Committee on Medical Education of the General Faculty*, Committee on Medical Education (October 31, 1950).

(Phase II), and the coordinator for clinical services (Phase III) have met with students immediately after a teaching program. Although this is not a new process in itself, the technique used had certain unique features. The coordinator of a program did not himself teach but supervised the educational program in the whole of the particular year or service. Thus his view was broad and his judgment reflected the purposes of the program. He chose eight to ten students at random to join him and discuss the immediately completed subject materials. Students soon found that it was not necessary to bring only criticism of a derogatory sort, but that positive suggestions which would enable the faculty to improve aspects of the syllabus, the laboratory, the lecture, or even the whole program, were welcome. Student response was recorded carefully by the coordinator and reported back to the teaching groups. Many changes resulted from these immediate critical sessions, and in general they were rich in content and truly reciprocal among students and coordinators. Although the changes were never made as fast as students hoped, they were progressive, real, and dependable.

Student Committee on Medical Education. Beginning with the second class under the revised program of medical education, Class of 1957, the Student Committee on Medical Education was formed, made up of volunteers from the class and two faculty advisers chosen by the students—one a preclinical scientist and one a clinician. This group met at intervals and participated in researches of their own choosing. They conducted surveys of their student colleagues, held meetings with faculty members, and wrote reports that were subsequently given to the Committee on Medical Education and to certain of the subject committees. This Student Committee on Medical Education continued for approximately eight years and was formally requested by the Committee on Medical Education of the faculty to prepare written reports each year to be circulated to the faculty and to be discussed at the annual meeting of the faculty. There is no doubt that this group had a very considerable influence on faculty thinking.

Then came some three or four years of doldrums when no activity of moment occurred. Three years ago, however, the students took the initiative to form again a Student Committee of Medical Education and to subdivide their activities into a variety of units, including curriculum, evaluation, and student affairs. There has been a resurgence of student enthusiasm and independent student initiative, with obvious increase in participation. Carefully formed questionnaires have been developed and circulated to the students. These have been submitted to research personnel on the faculty for comment so that their reliability could be high. The results have been discussed with the subject committees. In addition, students rated faculty members for their performance, and great dignity was shown in the transmission of these confidential materials to one person on the faculty by the students, namely, the chairman of the particular subject committee. The students have shown the same sense of responsibility to faculty as they as students wish shown to them.

Student Council. The Student Council has been a long-standing organizational unit, elected by each class, with class representatives coming together to take up matters of importance to students. The faculty has turned to the Student Council for representation on medical school committees. The Student Council has either recommended or held elections for members of the class to serve on faculty committees. For example, an elected representative for each of the first three classes now serves as a regular member of the Committee on Medical Education. That representation occurred for the first time in 1969. Thus a total of seventeen years was required for the students to become an integral part of the policy-making group of the general faculty. Students are also selected for the Medical School Committee on Student Affairs, and the Committee on Counseling, and they have taken the initiative in creating a curricular option of community medicine, have planned lecture series on their own, and have participated in student health projects.

There appears to be little doubt that we have now arrived at the point where the faculty is comfortable in working with students at a policy level in developing teaching methods and evaluation of instructional methods.

Responsible Participation of Students, Faculty, Administration, and Community as Colleagues

It is not enough to leave this presentation which is based so largely on the needs of the student without indicating appropriately the needs of the others with whom the student participates as a responsible colleague. Four peer groups are recognized, namely, the students themselves, the faculty, the administration, and the community, which in this case includes the patient. Each member has loyalty to his own group.

The faculty, during periods of enormous increase in knowledge, in the demands of science, in the requirements for patient care, and in changing patterns of teaching, must confer among themselves, but not wholly among themselves. Similarly, the administration, a support structure for both students and faculty, has its own needs as it attempts to find the necessary funds, equipment, facilities, and leadership to meet the prime objectives of a school of medicine. And then for the community—patients and others—the needs are of transcendent importance these days, as an attempt is made to distribute health services equally.

There is a grave danger that peer groups will remain separate, will treat their own problems, but will never really come to grips with those problems which require combined endeavor. However, as future demands become greater in many areas, the nature of the needs of each peer group may require that these groups come together, each keeping its identity, as they work as colleagues on mutual problems. This can be done; it is now being done; and it forms a basis for progress in solving problems.

University and Man

The question may well be asked, what is the object of the university that is truly universal? Certainly it is not the establishment of a campus, the design of a budget, or the creation of an administration in itself. It is not the gathering of huge funds from the federal government, the states, and the alumni for research, buildings, and endowment. The university is universal to man. By this I mean that the importance of man—his culture, his life, his role—is the central theme of the university. When this prime focus is obscured, the university itself becomes a series of confused academic specialties, each aimlessly functioning, each to some degree frustrated. With the increasing complexity that now challenges the university, the conflicts between unity of purpose and diversity of activities must be clarified. Weaver states the problem well, as follows: "The major thesis I will state is this: that as man controls his environment, giving him time to think and to make discoveries leading to further control, he has progressively uncovered more and more complications; but at the same time he has succeeded in discovering more and more unifying principles underlying unity. He has, in short, discovered the many and the one."[11]

Millis has presented the unity centering on man and the diversity of approaches that are central to the roles of the university.[12] We think of two major forces within the university. There are centrifugal forces of diversity, such as the powerful trusts of research, specialization in hundreds of fields, multiple departments, and separate schools of the university. Contributions by faculty experts in each area have advanced our knowledge and skills in an incalculable manner and continue to do so in geometric progression.

But contributing to unity is a centripetal force that allows us continuously to rediscover man. We find him in the person of the student, as the reason for education; in the teacher, as a guide for the student; in the patient, as the reason for medical care; and in the individual person, as the ultimate element of our local, national, and international communities.

The conflict between powerful centrifugal and centripetal forces can generate the kind of violent criticism that is heard when observers speak of science making man impersonal, specialization destroying recognition of the individual, research excluding teaching of the student, or automation destroying the teaching of the individ-

[11] W. Weaver, "Confessions of a Scientist-Humanist," *Saturday Review*, May 28, 1966, pp. 12–15.

[12] J. R. Millis, personal communication.

ual. Conversely, there is need for continuing movement in a dynamic equilibrium between the special field and the individual man. In this way, conflict is converted in symbiosis or mutual interdependence. This simplification of enormous complexity sets us free to plan changes based on excellence for man as well as for diverse fields. It is cooperative endeavor of peer groups who learn how to be responsible colleagues. The privilege of this clinical investigator looking at medical education has been the rediscovery of the medical student as a responsible colleague who will join in advancing medicine, in learning, in patient care, and in participating appropriately with other members of the university. The proper study of medicine is man.

ACKNOWLEDGMENT: Research for these studies was aided in part by a grant from the Commonwealth Fund of New York.

The Impact of New Discoveries on Medical Practice: Advances in the Diagnosis and Treatment of the Infectious Diseases

HARRY F. DOWLING, M.D.

Medical Consultant, the University of Delaware
Formerly Professor and Head of the Department of Medicine, the University of Illinois

I

HISTORY HAS BEEN CALLED "a nightmare" and "a dust heap." It has also been praised as "the world's court of judgment" and "the lamp by which our feet are guided." And both extremes are true. History may be nothing more than idle tales told to amuse the indolent, or it may be "philosophy teaching by examples," depending upon the uses to which it is put. I want to consider only a fragment of history and to put it to a modest use: to review briefly the recent progress in the diagnosis and treatment of the infectious diseases in the past fifty years and to show the effects of this progress upon the work of the practicing doctor.

Let us look back a few years. When the first *United States Pharmacopoeia* was published, in 1820, doctors were no longer giving a mixture of writing ink and cerebrospinal fluid for baldness, as the Egyptians did; nor the excreta of animals, as was common in the Middle Ages; yet this pharmacopoeia contained many therapeutically useless herbs, such as garlic and goldenrod, along with other preposterous substances like isinglass, cantharides, and lead. In the whole book I can find only twenty active drugs. Among these were three specifics for infections: quinine for malaria, mercury for syphilis, and ipecac for amebic dysentery. Other effective drugs were opium, belladonna, digitalis, and a few substances that either quieted the gastrointestinal tract or purged it. Well could Oliver Wendell Holmes say in 1860 that "if we throw out opium, the anesthetics and a few specifics, I firmly believe that if the whole materia medica, as now used, could be sunk to the bottom of the sea, it would be all the better for mankind—and all the worse for the fishes."

But the modern therapeutic era had already begun long before that. Its first landmark was the introduction into Europe, in the early eighteenth century, of the practice of inoculating with smallpox to prevent that disease, followed by Jenner's demonstration in 1798 that cowpox would do the same thing more safely. Laboratory research began to pay off in 1885 when Pasteur first used a laboratory-made vaccine to protect against rabies. These experiments paved the way for the many vaccines and serums in use today.

Meanwhile, chemical compounds had also proved to be potent magic bullets. The idea that if one looked hard enough, a chemical substance could be found which, when attached to a microorganism, would put it out of business, was at first only a glimmer in the mind of Paul Ehrlich. But by pursuing this idea he produced arsphenamine and neoarsphenamine, in 1909 and 1912 respectively. These became mainstays in the therapy of syphilis, until penicillin arrived.

The twenty years from 1912 until 1932, when the first of the sulfonamides was patented, seemed long to those who were caring for patients at the time, but in retrospect it was really a very short period, in comparison with the lack of progress in other centuries. And even this interval was punctuated by the synthesis of pamaquin and quinacrine for malaria in 1924 and 1930.

The story of the sulfonamides has been written many times: sulfanilamide was synthesized in 1908 and then put away on a shelf and forgotten. In 1913 Eisenberg showed that azo dyes had some effect against bacteria in the test tube. In 1932 Domagk found that one of these dyes, prontosil rubrum, protected animals from streptococcal infections. Soon thereafter, French investigators reported that the azo dye was not essential, that the effective component was sulfanilamide. Since this relatively simple substance was not patented, doctors all over the world were free to use it. More important still, chemists could modify it easily.

The first of these modifications was sulfapyridine. After it was developed in the pharmaceutical firm of May and Baker, Dr. Lionel Whitby showed that it was effective in pneumococcal infections in mice. When this success had been repeated in patients with pneumonia, one of the London newspapers headed a news article, "Thank you, Dr. Whitby." At the end of the next bacteriology lecture, the students rose as one body and shouted, "Thank you, Dr. Whitby."[1]

Were the students right? Who should get the credit for sulfapyridine? Should it be Gelmo who synthesized the parent compound, Eisenberg who showed its effectiveness in the test tube, Domagk who demonstrated this in animals, the group at the Pasteur Institute who identified the basic drug, the industrial chemists who modified the molecule to produce sulfapyridine, Whitby who showed its effectiveness in animals, or the clinicians who treated the first patients with pneumonia? The fallacy of honoring a single individual for the discovery of a new drug is nowhere better shown. Trying to cut the credit pie into properly sized slices recalls the words of the ancient preacher, "Vanity of vanities; all is vanity."

After several more effective and less toxic sulfa drugs were found, the vein of ore petered out in this field. But similar methods of chemical prospecting uncovered other drugs, an important one being isoniazid, the first chemical with practical effectiveness against tuberculosis. Even more significant from a scientific standpoint are three drugs which have a definite though limited effect in viral infections: idoxuridine, in the therapy of herpes simplex conjunctivitis, and methisazone and amantadine, prophylactics against smallpox and some influenza viruses, respectively. They hold out the promise

[1] Cyril Keele, "100 Years of Progress in the Drug Treatment," *Roy. Soc. Health J.* 83 (Nov.–Dec. 1963): 325–330.

of preventing or shortening other viral infections in the not-too-distant future.

Long before the antiviral drugs were available, the antibiotic era was well under way. Penicillin was discovered in 1929. Other important discoveries were streptomycin, the first effective antituberculosis agent, in 1944; chlortetracycline, the first broad-spectrum antibiotic, in 1948; and modifications of the penicillin molecule to make it active against additional bacteria, spotlighted by the introduction of methicillin in 1960.

II

So much for the bare bones of events as they occurred. How did these drugs affect the health of the people?

Mortality rates from scarlet fever, tuberculosis, typhoid fever, and dysentery had been declining for many decades before the advent of antibiotics or specific chemicals, as a result of improvements in personal hygiene, nutrition, and sanitation, and of changes in the virulence of microorganisms and the susceptibility of the population. Thus, we must not deceive ourselves that every favorable trend resulted from man's puny efforts. Dubos describes how Bombay rats have become resistant to plague and rabbits are becoming resistant to myxomatosis, and adds, ". . . if the rats and rabbits have a racial memory they may come to take pride in the illusion that it was through some conscious action of their own that they achieved control over the great epidemics of the past."[2]

Yet in spite of the complicated web of cause and effect, it is possible to trace the effects of man-made factors on some diseases. The best case for the lowering of death rates by chemotherapy and antibiotic therapy can be found among the respiratory diseases. It is unlikely that changes in living habits have diminished the spread of virulent bacteria by the respiratory route—if anything, the increased crowding of busy urban life would favor their spread. Thus, the fall in mortality rates for pneumonia and influenza from about 200 per 100,000 population in 1900 to about one-sixth that number, or

[2] René Dubos, *Mirage of Health* (Garden City, N.Y.: Doubleday and Co., 1961), p. 81.

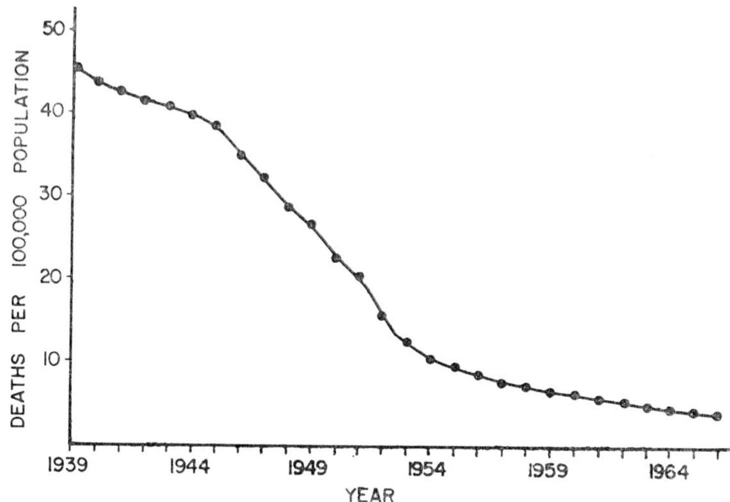

Mortality from tuberculosis, United States, 1939–1966.

31, for the years 1949 to 1951 appears to have resulted from serum, sulfonamide, and finally antibiotic therapy.[3]

Some years ago Lepper and I found that the fatality rate for patients who received no specific treatment was 30.5 per cent on our wards.[4] Treatment with specific serum decreased this to 16.9 per cent and sulfonamide treatment to 12.3 per cent, but neither was as effective as treatment with penicillin or the tetracyclines. Only 5.1 per cent of patients treated with these agents died, and the deaths were almost entirely in patients over the age of fifty years. But the fatality rate was still 15 per cent for patients over the age of sixty, with the best of treatment.

The effect of antimicrobial therapy can also be shown in tuberculosis (see figure above). The mortality rate declined slowly until 1944, but the sharp drop after that was almost certainly the result of the use of streptomycin and other antituberculosis agents.

[3] C. Dauer, R. F. Korns, and L. M. Schuman, *Infectious Diseases* (Cambridge, Mass.: Harvard University Press, 1968), p. 175.

[4] Harry F. Dowling and Mark H. Lepper, "The Effect of Antibiotics (Penicillin, Aureomycin, and Terramycin) on the Fatality Rate and Inci-

More direct evidence for the effectiveness of the newer drugs is seen in lowered case fatality rates for many diseases. Some of these are meningococcic meningitis, untreated, approximately 75 per cent, treated with sulfonamides or penicillin, 10 per cent; pneumococcic meningitis, untreated, approximately 100 per cent, treated with penicillin 30 per cent; tuberculosis meningitis, untreated, 100 per cent, treated with isoniazid, about 10 per cent; endocarditis caused by penicillin-sensitive streptococci, untreated, approximately 100 per cent, treated with penicillin and streptomycin, 5 per cent.

III

But the "wonder drugs" did not accomplish all this alone; they had a partner. Before the doctor uses a drug he must know what he is treating. Diagnosis, at least a tentative diagnosis, should precede therapy. Over the centuries the techniques of diagnosis have advanced progressively, but always less spectacularly than advances in therapy.

The information needed to diagnose infections can be divided into (1) general symptoms and signs of infection, (2) evidence of injury to a particular organ and of the extent of the damage, and (3) tests that show what microorganism is causing the infection. The doctor may make a tentative diagnosis from one or parts of all of these, but only by reasonably complete knowledge of all three can he make the best diagnosis, the one that ensures optimal therapy.

If we consider general signs, most patients with infection have fever and a rapid heart rate. The ancients detected these by observing the flushed face of the patient or feeling his hot skin and his pulse. Centuries passed before even the simplest instruments of precision were used. In 1707 a physician devised a "pulse-watch" which ran for one minute so that the heart rate could be counted.[5] This novel device did not catch on, and pulse-counting was not commonly practiced until the end of the nineteenth century. Similarly, the

---

dence of Complications in Pneumococcic Pneumonia: A Comparison with Other Methods of Therapy," *Amer. J. Med. Sc.* 222 (Oct. 1951): 396–403.

[5] Charles Singer and E. Ashworth Underwood, *A Short History of Medicine*, 2nd ed. (New York: Oxford University Press, 1962), p. 171.

earliest thermometers were too cumbersome to be used in patients; as late as 1870 a clinical thermometer exhibited before the British Medical Association was a foot long and an inch thick.[6]

After watches and thermometers, doctors added other procedures to detect infection. They learned that in many infections the number of leucocytes in the blood was increased and that the red blood cells, when placed in a tube, sedimented more rapidly than those of a normal person. But, on the whole, the information the doctor could obtain regarding general evidences of infection was minimal. Much more could be learned by detecting injury to particular organs.

Although the Greeks in the time of Hippocrates paid more attention to the general constitution of the patient, they also identified the organ involved in an infection by noting that it was red or swollen or emitted a discharge. They related jaundice to the liver. They placed their ears against the chest and heard the scraping sounds of pleurisy and the splash of air and fluid in the chest.

Little was added in the next two thousand years. In 1761 Auenbrugger described the difference in sounds following percussion of normal lungs and those containing a solid area of inflammation or covered by a layer of fluid. In 1819 Laennec reported that the sounds made by the lungs in breathing could be heard best through a tube, one end of which was applied to the chest and the other to the doctor's ear. Later this was modified into the double-tubed stethoscope which is seen today in every physician's pocket.

Yet percussion and auscultation sometimes failed even the most skilled doctors. In 1919 Sir William Osler, one of our greater physicians, died because none of the array of leading diagnosticians attending him detected the empyema that had formed over his pneumonia.

When X rays were discovered in 1895 they were first used to study bones and other solid objects; later they were employed effectively to detect abnormalities of the softer tissues, such as the lungs, liver, kidneys, spleen, and intestines. In recent years certain radioactive isotopes have been found to localize in certain organs. The

[6] J. Gershon-Cohen, "A Short History of Medical Thermometry," *Ann. New York Acad. Sc.* 121 (Oct. 9, 1964): 4–11.

rays emitted from these isotopes, impinging on a photographic plate, show the extent of the organ and leave a blank area where normal tissue has been replaced by products of disease.

One ingenious method of detecting local damage consists of demonstrating that injury to some organs results in an outpouring of certain enzymes into the blood. Today many different enzymes are measured to localize disease to particular organs and to determine the degree of damage.

One further example: Ever since asepsis became an accepted surgical technique, it has been feasible to cut out a small amount of tissue from the skin or from an internal organ, or to remove a lymph node. But only in recent years has this technique of biopsy (literally, "looking at living tissue") been practiced widely. Now it frequently becomes the final recourse when the doctor is not sure where the disease is located.

The third class of diagnostic procedures consists of those that detect the specific agent causing the disease. In some diseases, antibodies to the microorganism circulate in the blood after the first few days of infection. These can be detected by mixing the serum with the microorganism in the test tube.

In diagnosing other infections, a skin test is helpful. For instance, when an extract of tubercle bacilli is injected into the skin of a person who has had tuberculosis, it will cause redness and swelling at that site. In the past, when most people had tuberculosis in at least a mild form at some time in their lives, such a high percentage of people reacted positively to this test that it could not be used to diagnose the disease, except in young children. Today, when only a fraction of the population has ever had the disease, a positive tuberculin test usually means an active tuberculous infection.

The microorganism causing an infection is often identified, under the microscope, in a body fluid or tissue after staining with an appropriate dye. For example, American doctors in the 1890's frequently used the term "typho-malarial fever" to explain the serious febrile illnesses observed in the summer months, which we now know were two separate diseases, typhoid fever and malaria. Culture of the typhoid bacillus took a day or two, but the malarial parasite had been discovered in 1880 by Alphonse Laveran and could usually be seen in an unstained preparation of blood from a patient with malaria, if one looked long and hard enough. My former chief, Dr. Thomas Boggs, told me that The Johns Hopkins Hospital, around the turn of the century, set aside two wards each summer, one for typhoid fever and one for malaria. When a patient with fever was admitted without the signs of a local infection, he was held in an admitting ward until the intern had searched in the microscope for malarial parasites—for several hours if necessary! If they were not found, the patient was placed in the typhoid ward. Only by such crude and exhausting methods was the chief of that medical service able to state so positively: "Is there a typho-malarial fever? Yes, in the brains of doctors but not in the bodies of the patients."[7] Today, although both diseases are rare in the United States, techniques of staining malarial parasites assure a simpler, faster, and more accurate diagnosis, when the need arises.

Finally, the causative agent is determined unequivocally by culturing it. In tuberculosis, for instance, the culture is usually from the sputum, but if other organs are infected, the urine, or the cerebrospinal, pleural, or other fluid, or tissue from a biopsy, may yield the clinching diagnosis.

IV

Although I have discussed diagnosis and therapy separately, they are by no means unrelated. Rather, they advance hand in hand. Pneumonia is a good example. The pneumococcus, the microorganism that causes most pneumonias, was not discovered until 1886, half a century after Laennec's teachings had become established practice. This eventually led to the production of antiserums. Thus, diagnosing pneumococcal pneumonia was insufficient; the specific type of pneumococcus had to be identified. To this end, methods were perfected for growing pneumococci rapidly by inoculating sputum or blood into a mouse and mixing the peritoneal exudate with different serums, each containing antibodies against a single

[7] Harvey Cushing, *The Life of Sir William Osler* (New York: Oxford University Press, 1925), I, 446.

type. But even this took twelve to twenty-four hours, during which time the doctor was unable to give any effective therapy. Finally, in 1932, a rapid method was perfected, based on the swelling of the capsule of the pneumococcus when it was mixed with an antiserum specific for its type. This could give an answer in as short a time as fifteen minutes.

With the advent of the sulfonamides and penicillin, identifying the type of pneumococcus became unnecessary, since these drugs were effective against all types. Thus it is seen that obsolescence occurs in diagnostic procedures as well as in therapy.

The antibiotics provide another example of the interrelationship of diagnosis and therapy. Some strains of microorganisms are susceptible to an antibiotic and others are not. Consequently, it is often necessary to grow the microorganism in the presence of different concentrations of various antibiotics and then to select the antibiotic that inhibits the growth of that particular strain.

V

Now let us turn to results of these advances in diagnosis and therapy. What has been the effect of lowered mortality rates on the population? For one thing, they have reshuffled the age distribution. Average life expectancy was twenty-two years in ancient Rome; it was forty-nine years in the United States at the beginning of the twentieth century; and it is seventy years today. Thus we have in this country the problem of twenty million people over the age of sixty-five (whose medical expenses are only covered in part by Medicare) and the problem of increasing numbers of children and young people (which isn't solved at all by the Hippies). We also have the world-wide problem of increased starvation because of burgeoning populations.

On the bright side, most children can expect to live to a healthy old age. As late as the nineteenth century a family was fortunate if half their children lived to be adults. The difference between the despair of the past and the hopefulness of today is the difference between the lines of Pindar,

Life, the cheat, blows such a shifting gale
that none may keep the course he thinks to sail,

and the resounding words of the fifth chapter of Job,

Thou shalt come to thy grave in a full age,
like as a shock of corn cometh in the season.

Today parents can plan a life career for a child with reasonable confidence that he will live to carry it through. Planning for the future is no longer four futile words.

Second, the dread, the nameless terror, inspired by those things that men cannot understand and cannot control, was especially characteristic of epidemics during which men stood by hopelessly while families and whole towns were wiped out. We have heard a faint echo of this in recent years in the fear of poliomyelitis. But this degree of fear was artificially whipped up by a campaign for funds which stressed the crippling effects of the disease and said little about the thousands of persons who had no symptoms of illness, although they had become infected and developed immunity. These fears quickly passed when a vaccine became available, and at their height there was nothing to compare with the horror reflected in Poe's *Masque of the Red Death*, which describes a visitation of the plague. Of the three scourges of mankind—pestilence, famine, and war—we have the means to be practically free of the first two. The last we have not overcome.

Thirdly, I believe—and here I am sure to find critics—that the total sum of pain and discomfort from disease in this country is less than it was a hundred or even fifty years ago. The high fever and the sharp chest pain of pneumonia, for instance, are now usually over within a day after the doctor starts treatment, instead of being prolonged for a week or ten days and followed by an extended convalescence, if the patient recovered at all. Tuberculosis, instead of requiring confinement to bed for a year or two, often accompanied by frequent punctures of the chest wall to introduce air and collapse a lung, is now usually treated with drugs alone, while the patient is up and about, and he may be back at work in six months. The contrast rests between the pale but beautiful heroine of novel and opera, who slowly wasted away while preserving her glamor, and the healthy mother of four children for whom tuberculosis is an almost forgotten episode in the remote past.

VI

Finally, we come to the effect these changes have on the doctor's practice. Certain effects are obvious: although infectious diseases are still the most common of all illnesses, the patient usually gets well promptly after receiving the proper treatment, or has a mild disease which subsides without therapy.

On a typical day in 1866 (Table 1) Dr. John Burke, a practi-

TABLE 1: *Number of Patients Visited*

	New York City 1866	Decatur, Illinois 1950–1953
Pneumonia	1	70
Scarlet fever	2	0
Typhoid fever	4	0
Tuberculosis	2	0
Dysentery	1	0
Remittent fever	1	0
Peritonitis	1	0
Pericarditis	0	1
Meningococcic meningitis	0	1
Total, serious infections	12	72
Minor infections	9	469
Noninfectious diseases	3	459
Total	24	1,000

tioner in New York City, visited in their homes a total of twenty-four patients: two with scarlet fever, four with typhoid fever, one with pneumonia, two with tuberculosis, one with dysentery, one with remittent fever (probably malaria), one with peritonitis—all serious infections; nine others had less severe infections, and only three of the twenty-four had noninfectious illnesses.[8] In contrast,

[8] C. Rosenberg, "The Practice of Medicine in New York a Century Ago," *Bull. Hist. Med.* 41 (May–June 1967): 223–253.

among a thousand patients seen in their homes in Decatur, Illinois, nearly ninety years later, only 7 per cent had serious infections. Another 47 per cent had minor infections and 46 per cent had noninfectious diseases.[9]

Thus, the perplexing problems in a doctor's practice are now mostly among the noninfectious diseases. In the past, patients with chronic diseases often died when an acute infection occurred. The patient could not combat both the infection and the underlying disease. Today the new drugs often stop these infections each time they occur, and the patient lives on with his chronic disease. Also, the longer span of life enables people to live on into the age period where they develop diseases of the heart and blood vessels, chronic pulmonary disease, and cancer.

The increasing numbers of people with chronic diseases, and the twenty million over the age of sixty-five, have forced doctors to focus more attention on rehabilitation, the proper delivery of medical care, the problems of old age, and the emotional factors associated with illness. Although doctors are beginning to rise to the challenge, much remains to be learned and much to be done.

A second effect of recent advances in the diagnosis and therapy of infections has been the increase in the sheer volume of what a doctor needs to know. The medical profession went through a period of overdosing with drugs in the late eighteenth and the nineteenth centuries. This was followed by a period of therapeutic nihilism, especially among the medical leaders, in which the diagnosis was considered all-important and therapy was relegated to the background because there was so little one could do.

Physicians trained in the school of therapeutic nihilism were poorly equipped for the dozens of effective new drugs which appeared in the twentieth century. Because so few drugs had been effective in the past, doctors in general lacked the skills necessary to develop a critical attitude toward a new drug. Meantime, the deluge

[9] W. T. Couter, A. T. Held, and C. L. York, "Analysis of One Thousand Consecutive Residence Visits to Acutely Ill Medical Patients," *J.A.M.A.* 152 (Aug. 29, 1953): 1704–1706.

of advertising descended upon them, and the doctors were often swept along in the current.

Thus the medical profession lost a great opportunity. The bulk of the new remedies appeared first in the infectious-disease field. Had doctors learned how to understand them and use them well, they would have been able to cope with the successive waves of new drugs that appeared in other therapeutic areas.

In diagnosing and treating patients with their puzzling illnesses, doctors are like troops in the front lines. Although medical scientists are continually developing new weapons for the war against disease, among the most important of which are new drugs, these weapons are worthless unless the soldiers understand them and know how to use them. Only by becoming familiar with the new drugs as they are put in his hands can the practicing doctor keep the mortality rates from pneumonia, tuberculosis, meningitis, and a host of other diseases as low as they are. He can be helped by journals, textbooks, postgraduate education, computer systems, and television beamed into his office, but he alone has the responsibility of learning and staying abreast, and this is a tremendous job in itself.

Third, when the newer drugs are used, diagnosis and treatment often require special skills and complex apparatus. This has meant that a higher proportion of patients must be treated in hospitals where the skilled people and the apparatus can be mobilized. Admissions to hospitals for acute illnesses rose from 59 per 1,000 population in 1935 to 136 per 1,000—more than twice as many—in 1960.[10]

Finally, the practice of the physician has been changed in a more subtle way by the new discoveries in infectious diseases. People today do not expect to die of an infection; they know that many nonlethal infections can be quickly checked, and they look forward to a long life, essentially free from serious disability. Their hopes are high—sometimes too high. The patient holds his doctor in high esteem and is willing to follow the doctor's orders, confident that

[10] Monroe Lerner and Odin W. Anderson, *Health Progress in the United States, 1900–1960: A Report of the Health Information Foundation* (Chicago: University of Chicago Press, 1963), pp. 246–247.

he can see the gold at the end of the rainbow. But when the patient fails to get well promptly, the doctor's image is quickly tarnished. Thus, in the few serious infections that are yet unsolved, such as infectious hepatitis or encephalitis, and in the many non-infectious diseases for which we can at present do little, the patient or his family may expect a cure when there is none. Fortunately, most people can accept the fact that the secret of immortality has not yet been given to doctors or anyone else. But though we may never reach this goal, we can come closer to achieving for everyone a life which is happy and healthy, until the infirmities of age make it necessary that he move on and give place to someone else.

Centuries ago the prophet said, "Your old men shall dream dreams, your young men shall see visions." To those who are my age it is pleasant to look back on the conquests of the last few decades, to contrast today's plethora of remedies with yesterday's scarcity, and to have seen, at first hand, what this change has meant to people's lives. But what to us are dreams of the past are to the younger men and women today visions of what is yet to come. I hope that they may have heard, in the stories of the giants of the past, the clear call, "Go thou and do likewise."

Changing Concepts of Deviance

DOUGLAS D. BOND, M.D.

Case Western Reserve University
Cleveland, Ohio

ALTHOUGH I WAS SUPPOSED to give some kind of history of psychiatry, I felt that anyone interested in that subject could read about it in standard texts and learn its history from far better authorities than myself. What seemed to me more interesting was to examine the whole perspective of deviance in general, and what is called "illness," for illness exemplifies a certain kind of deviance, or, perhaps more accurately, a certain way of looking at deviance.

If we talk about deviant behavior we must have some concept of a norm from which to deviate; yet normality is a tricky concept for which our definitions are neither cogent nor firm. We can have practical definitions, so that if someone says he feels fine, and he looks all right to us, we say he is normal. This has a lot of practical but very little theoretical value. Certainly the definition of "normal" has changed as knowledge of the workings of the body has increased. For example, we now signify changes in cells as abnormal or deviant, when only a very few years ago we would never even have thought of examining them. To define health we must think of certain balances that maintain the safety of the organism, protect its life, and provide for the fullest use of its various functional capacities. In this framework all illness tends to hamper or threaten the organism's existence or functional capacity.

Health, or the normal, has never been of much interest to physicians. It has always seemed dull, merely the absence of disease—and if one questions a physician who has just examined a patient with no "positive" findings, he will say that the patient has "nothing." Even the word *positive* is peculiar here, but so accustomed are we to search for disease that to change the word to *negative* would be a wrench. This disease orientation of the physician has had great advantages. The imbalance brought by disease to the functioning of the organism has been used as a window through which to see the balance of health. Where would medicine—or indeed biology—be, had we surveyed the size of livers, say, and concluded that some people have big livers, some small, and some medium sized, and that this is the natural distribution. Such a concept of natural distribution carries with it a tacit set of acceptance or of inevitability. The concept of pathology, of disease, of something that is wrong and should be changed has been basic to medicine, to research, and to treatment.

This whole disease orientation is now under attack. The physician is condemned for its narrowness and many people want something more—something in the area of increasing potential or increasing happiness. In biology we have certainly moved beyond the need for an illness which one can view as an experiment of nature—to point the way for the investigator. The direct approach in the biochemical and biophysical mechanisms in the organism is now at hand and direct intrusion into the mechanisms will prove infinitely fruitful. But before we leave the subject of disease orientation, I would like to point out that Pauling's Nobel Prize in chemistry came because of interest in two diseases—sickle-cell anemia, a common illness, and paroxysmal nocturnal hemoglobinuria, a most uncommon one—but these two illnesses led to the most fundamental discoveries on the shape and structure of the hemoglobin molecule.

A new generation of physicians will have a different and more modern outlook. We have certainly crossed a barrier, and when we now do research on the aging process, we can get grants to study it and, we hope, to cure it. What brave new world do we enter here? Will it be normal someday to reach only a certain age, or a certain height, to be a certain color? Will the increase in control that scientific knowledge gives tend to standardize us—to narrow the spectrum of what we now think of as normal? Can we stand these decisions? What constant controversy could obtain when the possibility of control is further realized? Man was spared decision and controversy when superstition reigned and it was the "gods" or nature who determined practically the whole environment and also man himself. If, however, we could exercise control, what arguments one could have with one's wife, parents, and in-laws over the ultimate size, color, sex, and IQ of a blessed event!

The maintenance of life and functional capacity demands an adaptation to the environment because no living thing is self-sufficient. It always takes from and gives to the environment. In physical terms the lack of adaptation leads to death. Let us look at the mental and the social sides.

If we have a hard time with the concept of physical health, we certainly have a worse one with mental and emotional health. We can see much the same dilemmas in definition and we see even hazier borders. But if we go about our definitions in the same way, we may get somewhere. To be normal mentally for one's age there are certain prerequisites. One must have some understanding of the world outside which we call reality. The concept of reality varies with the culture and with our understanding of it, but, nonetheless, one cannot be normal or be able to adapt without a grasp of it. Once we have some grasp of the reality outside ourselves, then some kind of adaptation is absolutely necessary to become self-sufficient and to be able to care for ourselves. We can see that the most difficult part of this environment to which we must adapt is other men. We can see that there are certain requirements in the environment for the adaptation to be normal. Adaptation to such an environment as a concentration camp or a prison might be heroic for a spell, but quite abnormal if it were preferred. In other words, the environment must provide the opportunity for the full use of one's mental capacities and the satisfaction of one's emotional drives, or it would be as restrictive on the mental sphere as the desert to a water bird.

If one were to characterize the role of psychiatrist, psychologist, social worker, or physician in past years, it would be to say that each of them worked to get someone who is out of step with society back into it, to help him adapt to it. This is not the same as to conform to it. Now the young and the disenchanted are saying, "Examine your environment. You will find that *it* is sick, not the people who refuse or cannot adapt to it." Replace your efforts at trying to adjust the individual to this sick society by social action that will modify the society, to better fit the requirements of individuals.

There is nothing new here except that, because of our modern science and medicine, the problem enters the health field in a philosophical way. Every great political and religious movement had some environmental change in mind. The various communist revolutions have all had, at their core, change in the human environment to enhance the hope of individual realization and opportunity. The tremendous revolution in labor practices, won in the last thirty-five years, has changed the lives of millions for the better.

At the interface of society and the mental functioning of the individual there is a new and confusing twist within our scientific attitude which inquires into the cause of things and the relationship between forces. We have undermined an older moral view. This conflict gives many of us great concern and is at the heart of much of our turbulence. Not long ago, the whole idea of free will and individual moral responsibility was widely held and, indeed, it underlies most of our legal foundations and social processes. It is based on church law, from which civil law was derived, and it is basically an attitude that a great many people still hold. The idea is simple—namely, that an individual knows right from wrong and is responsible for his actions. It was and is a simplistic view. There were no exceptions to this rule at first; then, only those persons who were most deviant were excepted, those who were deviant in that they did not see reality at all the way others did. This general state of things obtained with a certain general satisfaction, until recently. Now there is an explosion of discontent and disorder in this area. Under the impact of psychoanalysis, modern psychology, and sociology, the idea of individual responsibility has lessened and a kind of determination has taken hold. It is interesting that the assassination of Robert Kennedy, for instance, has met with a sadness, but no great public outcry for revenge. As Sirhan Sirhan's own personal history unfolds, one sees a miserable little boy, a brutal father, and great adversity. One compounds these into some kind of partial explanation that does not whet the appetite for revenge, but simply reveals another tragedy.

Following a similar path, alcoholism has been graduated from a moral defect to an illness. An illness in this instance is a deviance one cannot help. Not long ago an unmarried girl having her second abortion was considered a psychopath (i.e., a "bad" girl); now she is more likely to be looked upon as having suffered from two traumatic experiences. In these examples it is clear that we are moving away from moral judgments toward explanations for behavior that put the individual more in the position of victim than of perpetrator.

The opposition to this modern trend has its rational base in the fear that lack of individual accountability for one's action is a degrading influence on individuals and on society as a whole. There are always cases that cause public ire (e.g., when there is no question about the act, but the defendant is judged not guilty by reason of insanity). In this instance, the law, as I see it, turns a partial explanation for the behavior into an excuse. The law says, in effect, this man or woman's deviance is so great that he or she can no longer be held morally accountable for any action.

As knowledge about the formation of men's minds increases, we see greater complexity, particularly in the interplay between environment and the growing mind of the developing individual. It is exactly analogous to the tremendous increase in understanding and complexity that biochemical advances have brought in knowledge of the body. And just as these advances have made a quick definition of health impossible, so has knowledge of the developing mind shown the complexities in the determination of behavior, so that a quick differentiation of "normal" cannot be simplistic. To ask if someone at a given moment in the past knew right from wrong and was able to adhere to the right sounds simple, but to answer in an honest and intelligent way is almost always impossible. Our minds are too complex and too inconsistent.

It seems to me we have a major dilemma here, yet one that can be solved if we approach it properly. We should separate the concepts of explanation and excuse. For instance, there may be many reasons which determine, or at least partially determine, a man's act when the act is detrimental to society and therefore should be discouraged. I know a woman who shot an eight-year-old neighbor through the head, buried the gun in some hamburger meat in the freezer, dumped the body in a field, and then went shopping. A large number of people asked me, "Is there anything wrong with Mrs. C.?" The only answer I could give was "How normal can you be?" The act itself, in a case like this, speaks more loudly for senseless deviant behavior than anything one could find out about it. The verdict of "not guilty because of insanity" in Mrs. C.'s case does not sit well with any of us. In her instance "guilty because of insanity" would make more sense. The depth of the moral penetration into our legal system is clear here because it literally maintains that if you had no moral responsibility for the act by reason of derangement, you in effect did not commit the act.

I talk here of an extreme of deviant behavior, which showed its abnormality by being determined not by an external provocation from reality, but by distorted inner drives unmodified by a grasp on reality. It may be true that environmental pressures in the distant past were influential in distorting these drives, but if so, they were important in the developmental process.

Let us turn to deviants who are more obviously influenced by the society around them. How a society handles and even identifies such deviants is an important hallmark of that society. We probably delude ourselves into thinking that times are very different, in ways in which they are not. For instance, students' protests and riots are as old as universities. Student demand for authority started at least as far back as the Middle Ages when students *were* the authority. In both Spain and Italy universities grew out of bands of students who hired men to teach them and fired them when they were displeased. In the Middle Ages, riots of students in England and Paris progressed to pitched battles in which multiple deaths occurred on each side.

We had hoped we had moved to gentler times. With the great

growth in knowledge that has taken place in this country, particularly in science, and with the tremendous increase in population and the increased demand to go to universities, we have had to evolve a more complex structure. This structure is now seriously threatened by student criticism and questioning and the active support by many faculty—most of them young. Although many of these criticisms are rational and just—for our structures, like all structures, have become encrusted—there is great danger that the impatience and sharpness of the demands may make disappear much that is good. In the excitement of this mounting battle extraneous motives are included: the working out, or at least the expression, of personal hatreds toward authority that arise from attitudes toward one's parents; the simple excitement of battle; and the support of some cause, no matter what, that can bring the shy and the lonely an excuse for companionship. Again, there is the tendency to move responsibility for failure one step away from oneself. It is becoming increasingly popular to say that the student does not fail—the school fails. The man does not fail, society fails; and in a recent *Time* an English psychiatrist is quoted as saying that mental patients are not sick—society is sick.

It is a reversal of what we had taken as obvious before. We are merely saying now that it is up to a school to see that a student is happy and successful; up to society to ensure success. The conservatives among us have a point. Is it not degrading to remove all sense of personal responsibility? Does it not remove a valuable pride if one has to say of one's success, "The school did it—society did it—not I"? But the conservatives have gone too far in the past. Starvation is no incentive—hunger may be. The interweaving complexities of our society no longer leave any one of us "free" in the old sense. Prejudice against a man's skin, nationality, or religion still takes a horrible toll and this must be fought. Societal changes that move toward fairness are the good things that our protesters are protesting for.

The deviant serves us well here. The man or woman, girl or boy, who defies convention, who moves out of the Establishment to look at it with personal courage and clarity, may save us from perpetuating the wrongs that have gone before. But the older ones of us, who are, I suppose, members of the Established, wish the young reformers would realize that some of us once were young reformers, that we are not personally responsible for the world as it is. We inherited a good part of it and we have been tolerant enough to let the young have their strident say. I hope they realize also that the deviant's tragedy is success, because with success, which means a following, he is no longer deviant.

In the handling of deviants a society brands itself. A society that demands conformity stagnates, at best. A society that allows destructive deviation destroys itself. We try to find our way between. We seem to have an inertial force in society that swings to excessive motion, first one way, then another; yet it is the middle ground we seek. At this time we are more or less at a loss in our control mechanisms which we used to think were firm. To whom do we go to deal with the educational problems in our cities? For all kinds of services? Our demand for service has far outreached our supply, and the demands of men seem to have an infinite capacity to grow; our welfare and social systems are hopelessly inadequate; our teacher supply, in quantity and quality, is hardly better; our courts and the availability of legal services come nowhere near the need; the distribution of medical care is hardly better; even the distribution of food in this country of plenty leaves shocking pockets of starvation.

These defects demand solution—but how? The deviant fixes on the weak points in the Establishment and forces attention on them, perhaps too shrilly, but he does know the enormous inertia to change, and thus he pushes hard; harder and far more impolitely than many of us wish. The danger he faces is that he must gauge the strength and speed of his demand or he will create a counterforce against himself. He already has the conscience of the Established on his side and, once pricked, it can be a strong force. But no one likes looking for too long at his own conscience. I hope we can manage this dilemma so that reforms may come with deliberate speed, with acceptance of the need to act, and without the violence born of frustration.

Tempers are becoming short on both sides. This is not a good sign. We must pay attention to our methods. They are our safeguards. The only difference between a democracy and a totalitarian government is the methods that are used. Freedom of speech has to do fundamentally with the freedom to express ideas. We should be careful that it does not encompass too readily sheer invective or character assassination. The use of force for either repression or revolution is a dangerous tool; for force breeds counterforce, and that breeds war. Revolutions have been wrought in the thinking of men, without force. Jesus Christ, Gandhi, Martin Luther King are examples. Exercise of true force can bring revolution. Nazi Germany, Russia, China, and Cuba are examples—perhaps our own country, at its founding, is another, but that is a long time ago now.

If we are going to progress, we must all know that change is not always progress, that men still have the capacity for evil or destruction, and that adherence to the method in which debate and compromise, though heated, may be softened by reason is still the steady road to improvement. But it is enormously important that motion be evident in the right direction, for, as President Kennedy said in his inaugural address, "Those who oppose peaceful revolution make violent revolution inevitable!"

I have tried to speak of deviance in a very broad context. It is a concept that deserves broad treatment and one in which stereotypes need to be shaken. I have tried to make three points: (1) Concepts of health and disease are changing; and as we move toward a detailed interest in the biological process and the mechanisms that control it, we see that our older classifications are too rigid and too simple. We have been caught up in the intricacies of cause and effect and in the descriptive, almost moral judgment of health and disease—with illness as "bad" and health as "good." Furthermore, this increasing control over our lives will provide us with more and more complex decisions. (2) This same kind of thinking has penetrated to the mental and emotional sphere, due, in the beginning, I believe, to psychoanalytic findings. Here we have an even more revolutionary problem. Because of the original moral base of our law and the assumption of individual free will and moral responsibility, the discovery of a host of genetic and environmental factors in the development of an individual and his behavior has led us into the trap of regarding an explanation of behavior as an excuse for it. These concepts must be separated. Society must deter certain actions, regardless of their origin or the degree of our understanding. (3) Because it is an exaggeration, deviance from the usual permits us to learn much about the more hidden balances of homeostasis and the workings of the biological organism and its adaptation to its environment. We have learned, as well, many of the requirements for prolonging life and protecting it against the agents that threaten it.

The Development of Scientific Medicine

LESTER S. KING, M.D.

Senior Editor, Journal of the American Medical Association
Professorial Lecturer in the History of Medicine
University of Chicago

WHAT IS SCIENTIFIC MEDICINE? For some observers the scientific aspect of medicine lies in the truly awesome equipment that overflows our hospitals, laboratories, and doctors' offices. The dials and tubes seem to scream out a scientific pedigree. They render possible the innumerable tests to which the patients are subjected—the x-rays, blood chemistries, "scans," and the like, which provide accurate information. In the old days, when the physician relied on his unaided senses, he could only guess. But now with his instruments he can record with considerable accuracy what is going on inside the body, inside the individual organs, inside the cells; and these readings and results give a feeling of precision to both doctor and patient. This precision, for some, represents the scientific dimension of medicine.

Others equate scientific medicine with the ability to *do* something for a patient. Today the practicing physician has enormous power. He has at his command an outstanding array of remedies, and the greenest intern today performs acts of therapeutic skill far beyond the ability of an Osler. Scientific medicine, in this viewpoint, would be the capacity to bring about therapeutic triumphs.

But there is also a quite different view, that scientific medicine should refer to the ultimate goal of enlarging total medical knowledge, to asking questions of nature, questions of health and disease, and to finding out the answers. Curing the patient would then be only secondary; the primary aim would be knowledge for its own sake, regardless of its usefulness. And the goal of accumulating knowledge is distinctly different from that of curing a particular patient.

Although these two views represent vastly different attitudes, there is no necessary contradiction between them. We simply recognize a distinction between abstract knowledge and concrete application. One aspect of medicine looks toward the individual patient, to get him well from his particular disease. The other looks not at the individual patient but to knowledge in the abstract, to generalizations, to what in a previous generation was blandly known as the "laws of nature." And in all this, wherein lies science?

In seeking an answer to this question I would emphasize first of all that precision alone does not confer scientific value, and, second, that science does not deal with any individual fact or individual patient *considered in isolation*. If, say, a patient is very obese, weighing approximately 350 pounds, this isolated fact has no scientific value and precise measurement to the second decimal would not make the fact any more scientific. Let us say that the patient who weighed 350 pounds died at the age of 40. If we find that he died at the age of 40 years, 3 months, and 17 days, this added precision would not make our information more scientific. But suppose we look around us and find a number of comparable cases, then we might be willing to make a generalization and say that persons who are substantially overweight tend to die young, or, at least, younger than those who are slender. When we do this, we no longer consider the fact of obesity in isolation. We connect the obesity with something else—in this instance with early death. We assert a connection between the observation "obesity" and the observation "early death." The patient's 350 pounds are a fact. His death at the age of 40 is a fact. We believe there is some connection between them and we emphasize the connection when we make the general statement, "Fat people die earlier than thin people."

This statement may or may not be true, but that is a totally different question. True or not, the observation was first made by Hippocrates, some 2,300 years ago. In the work known as *The Aphorisms* he declared, "Persons who are naturally very fat are apt to die earlier than those who are slender."[1]

Fat people, like everyone else, exhibit an infinite number of different features. Hippocrates paid attention not to the color or the height of the fat people, nor to their parents, nor their diet, nor their skin or liver or thyroid, but only to the age they attained. Of all the infinite properties that apply to fat people, he abstracted one property for consideration, ignored all others, and then made a generalization. He asserted a roughly inverse relationship between weight and longevity. He identified a pattern in nature, a connection between apparently isolated facts, and, so far as we know, was the first one to perceive a relationship between these apparently disconnected data. The first stage of scientific medicine is the perception of relationships or patterns.

Hippocrates wrote down a large number of aphorisms. Let me mention a few: "Spasm supervening on a wound is fatal";[2] "In a pregnant woman, if the breasts suddenly lose their fullness, she has a miscarriage";[3] "In dropsical persons, ulcers forming in the body are not easily healed."[4] There are hundreds of others. Each of them represents a pattern of events, a clustering of phenomena, as if drawn together by some inner thread.

In another famous Hippocratic work, the *Prognostics* or *Prognosis*, he described certain signs, indicated what they meant, and predicted what was going to happen in the future. Let me give an example. "Children are likely to have convulsions if the fever is high . . . This most commonly happens in children under the age of

[1] Hippocrates, "Aphorisms" (Sec. 2, par. 44), in *The Genuine Works of Hippocrates*, trans. Francis Adams (Baltimore: Williams & Wilkins, 1939), p. 298.

[2] *Ibid.* (Sec. 5, par. 2), p. 308.

[3] *Ibid.* (Sec. 5, par. 37), p. 310.

[4] *Ibid.* (Sec. 6, par. 8), p. 314.

seven. As they grow up and reach adult years, they are no longer likely to be attacked by convulsions in the course of a fever, unless . . . in inflammation of the brain."[5]

He perceived a sort of pattern, a relationship between childhood and fevers and convulsions, with intrinsic connections between the separate terms. What the connections were he did not say. Just how fever was related to the convulsion and to childhood he did not know, nor why the tendency to convulsions decreased as the child grew up. In these texts, he merely asserted what his experience had taught him, that if he saw thus-and-so, then such-and-such would result. He was making predictions, and we all know that successful prediction is one of the hallmarks of good science. Hippocrates embodied his experience in writings that have persisted over 2,300 years, and during most of that time have guided physicians in their practice.

These aphorisms and prognostic declarations are, in essence, "rules of thumb," like the rules drawn from past experience which guide the good cook or the good farmer. Such rules not only declare what happened in the past, but also indicate what we might expect in the future.

Now for the moment let us compare medicine with some other activity—cooking, for example. A good cook can provide a set of directions telling what to do, but cannot ordinarily give a reason for doing one thing rather than another—except the very important reason that "it works." Cookbook directions furnish practical rules, without theoretical justification. They provide an excellent example of what is commonly known as empiricism. The empiricist knows that doing things in a particular way will bring about particular results, and he has formulated general rules derived from experience. But experience alone does not tell us much about the reasons behind a given activity, the rationale for a particular procedure, the *cause* of one or another phenomenon.

[5] Hippocrates, "Prognosis" (Sec. 24), in *The Medical Works of Hippocrates*, trans. John Chadwick and W. N. Mann (Oxford: Blackwell Scientific Publications, 1950), p. 127.

In contrast to the good practical cook, we have the person we may call the nutritional scientist who knows all the caloric values and the chemical composition of foods, the various reactions they undergo, and the physiological effects they induce. With such knowledge the nutritionist can explain why we mix the ingredients in order, what components must be measured carefully, why a particular oven temperature is necessary, what diets may be best for particular diseases. But the person with all this knowledge may or may not be able to prepare a decent, edible dinner. The good cook and the good nutritionist represent two distinct aspects of cooking.

The nutritionist, who can explain phenomena and supply the reasons why, exemplifies the rationalistic approach. Philosophy has long emphasized the rather sharp distinction between empiricism and rationalism, a distinction which was important in the days of Plato and Aristotle and is equally important today, a distinction that applies equally to cooking and to medicine.

Hippocrates exhibits a high order of empiricism. He furnished generalizations drawn from experience, quite comparable to the directions in the cookbook. But if we ask, Do these aphorisms constitute medical science? the answer would be No. They furnish what in essence is only the raw material of science.

Science must know the reasons why things happen, must know things by their causes, must offer explanations. When Hippocrates said, "Spasm supervening on a wound is fatal," the scientist wants to know *why*? How can you explain it? In other words, what is the *cause*? Hippocrates indicated three factors—the wound, the stiffness, and the fatal outcome. But not all wounds result in stiffness or death. Stiffness—today we would say *spasm*—can occur without a wound, and also without death. However, as Hippocrates validly asserted, a connection between these three elements does occur *under certain circumstances*. Under particular conditions, the nature of which was not clear to him, wounds and spasm seemed to go together, and this conjunction usually led to death. How to explain the conjunction was beyond his knowledge.

Modern medicine has clarified the reasons why the three factors sometimes coincide and sometimes do not. We now can tie together the separate phenomena—the wound, the stiffness, and the death—through an intermediate concept that we call infection, more precisely, infection with a specific organism called the tetanus bacillus. This new concept relates the separate data and shows them to be a logical part of an orderly pattern. To explain the phenomenon that Hippocrates described, we say that the wound became infected with tetanus spores, with eventual production of a toxin that attacked the nervous system and induced the spasm. We thus have provided "causal" factors. We can explain why, if a person has a wound, it may lead to spasm and death.

Hippocrates had noted certain individual facts and indicated that somehow they belonged together in a particular pattern. This was an empirical correlation. The concept of a specific infection, however, furnishes a rational dimension. It indicates the connecting links which tie together the empirical observations, like an underwater tunnel connecting the two banks of a river.

In his *Aphorisms* Hippocrates was content merely to indicate empirical correlations between events. In other writings, however, he did offer explanations by means of theoretical concepts, and the study of these is a major part of medical history. The explanations that Hippocrates used have no relation to such present-day concepts as infection, hypersensitivity, neoplasia, and the like. Instead, he used such terms as the so-called four humors—the blood, phlegm, yellow bile, and black bile. At times he spoke also of elements and qualities. In health there was a certain suitable proportion. If the proportion or harmony were disturbed, then a dyscrasia resulted, that is, an improper mixture, and this constituted disease.

If one humor became unduly preponderant, then disease was the consequence. A simple example, one that we can readily appreciate today, would be the common cold, a disease in which we have a runny nose. For Hippocrates the explanation would be an excess of phlegm in the body; the excess ran off through the nose. When proper proportion between the phlegm and the other three humors was restored, then the patient would return to health. Today we would say, using rather loose terminology, that the *cause* of the cold was a virus. For Hippocrates the cause was a disproportion of humors with an excess of phlegm.

Medical science must provide explanation for disease, find out causes, show the interconnections among the phenomena about us. The empiricist sees the surface of things. He notes that certain observations go together. The rationalist tries to see below the surface and discern the hidden forces that bring about the phenomena.

Over the centuries physicians have given a great many reasons *why* things happened and have offered a great many concepts to explain disease. We have had the humors and the faculties, the ferments, the excess of acid over alkali, the action of acrids, the mechanical blockage of tubules, an all-pervading gastroenteritis, infection by living agents—these represent only a few of the important explanations that have been offered at one or another time. The scientist continually tries to answer the questions Why? and How? and In what way? and the medical scientist tries to answer these questions in relation to disease.

When we study the history of medicine and the development of explanatory concepts, we must at all costs avoid the fallacy known as presentism—that is, judging or evaluating past doctrines by present standards. The past must be studied in its own context. The electron microscope and the discoveries to which it gives rise, as well as the new concepts that are engendered thereby, are all irrelevant when we study the achievements of Virchow. Equally irrelevant is our knowledge of microbiology when we study Benjamin Rush or William Cullen.

Galen, the greatest physician of antiquity, happened to be wrong in almost everything he said. But this shows not that he was a scientific ignoramus, but that the scientific concepts and standards of the second century were vastly different from those of the twentieth. The historian, to appreciate the scientific stature of Galen, must study him in his own intellectual environment, against the philosophic and cultural background of his own era, with its own presuppositions and attitudes. Galen made new observations, drew new inferences, and synthesized a body of knowledge that marked a great advance in medical science.

Of course, science does not stand still. Change, perhaps even progress, constantly takes place, not only in techniques and observations but in attitudes and in methodology and cultural trends. We must not isolate medical practice and medical science from their intellectual, social, and cultural environments. The historian of science, the historian of ideas, must reconstruct the past so that older doctrines and theories are displayed in a suitable perspective. Then, changes in doctrine will be seen to have their counterparts in other, broader changes. Indeed, the history of science will reflect, in a sense, the successive social, cultural, and intellectual transformations of mankind. To understand scientific medicine, we must keep in mind the intellectual background and its successive changes and development.

In line with this concept I would suggest two separate approaches to the study of medical history. For any given historical period we can take up the interrelationships between medical theory and the scientific views of that particular time. We can also take up the methodology of medicine, by which I mean the degree of critical acumen it shows, and see how this reflects the contemporary culture. Let me indicate some examples of each in turn, and their relevance to scientific medicine.

First I would like to present some relationships between chemistry and medicine. In the seventeenth century chemistry was making rapid progress, and some basic chemical reactions were carefully studied. Such investigators as van Helmont, Libavius, Glauber, Lemery, Tachenius, and, of course, Boyle laid the groundwork for modern chemistry and did so through experiments. These were as precise as the available techniques permitted. By modern standards the techniques were abysmally crude, but this is an ex post facto judgment, quite irrelevant to the merits of the investigators. The differences between acids and alkalis, their modes of preparation, the formation and decomposition of salts, the process of neutralization, the techniques of distillation, the phenomena of fermentation received a great deal of attention in the laboratory. And physicians—many of whom were capable chemists—began to use the concepts of chemistry to explain physiological phenomena. This was the movement known as iatrochemistry, vastly important in the history of medicine.

A leader of the iatrochemical movement was Franciscus Sylvius, who lived from 1614 to 1672.[6] He was primarily a clinician rather than an experimentalist, but he did adopt the chemical data of others and apply them to problems in medicine, both theoretical and practical. He believed that the fundamental chemical reaction in the body was the interaction between alkali and acid, particularly between the bile, which he considered alkaline, and the pancreatic juice, which he regarded as acid. The precise details were rather complicated and I have discussed them in considerable detail in the reference cited. Here I wish to comment on the processes of inflammation and ulceration.

The characteristics of inflammation were well known to ancient physicians, and the terms *rubor*, *dolor*, *tumor*, and *calor*, well described by Celsus, have regularly reappeared in medical textbooks since then. But how to *explain* these phenomena? How to proceed from a simple observational or descriptive approach to a scientific one? Sylvius tried to explain inflammation and ulceration by the action of acids and alkalis. Acids, for example, were "sharp." If applied to the tongue, they had a "bite." Sylvius believed that acid particles normally present in the blood could localize in a given area and, by virtue of their "sharpness," could produce the inflammation and, if sufficiently severe, an ulceration or erosion. To these sharp, eroding particles he gave the name of "acrids," and he distinguished acid and alkaline particles, each having the powers of erosion.

Sylvius "explained" various inflammatory states by attributing them to the local accumulation and action of corrosive particles. Proper therapy followed logically. If inflammation were due to a

[6] I have discussed the works of Sylvius at length in my recent book, *The Road to Medical Enlightenment, 1650–1695* (London: Macdonald; New York: American Elsevier, 1970).

local excess of acid, the appropriate remedy, clearly, would be the administration of alkali. If a local excess of alkali were the responsible factor, the physician should prescribe acid.

All this is completely logical and furnishes an elegant explanation for observed phenomena. There is, however, a major and to us rather obvious drawback—the evidence for the so-called acrids is quite indirect and rests on analogy. Sylvius had seen acids and alkalis in the retort, but he had not actually seen the acrids in the body. He had not demonstrated their presence in areas of inflammation. Even if acids and alkalis in the test tube and retort were quite familiar, the body is not a retort, a blood vessel not a test tube. Sylvius and his many followers were pursuing an analogy. Acids, when studied in the laboratory, obviously *can* erode, and the body *does* contain acid substances. Sylvius merely assumed that inflammation or ulceration occurring "spontaneously" in the body resulted from the action of acids that were present in the body.

Behind this view lay the whole humoral tradition of two thousand years, the tradition that long antedated modern chemistry, namely, that the body contains humors of varying properties. The concept that an acid humor could act in the body harmonized with the old as well as the new. Related to this was a further concept that a suitable balance, or proportion, must exist between different humors, and that an excessive quantity of one humor could induce disease. Hippocrates knew nothing of acids and alkalis, but he did know a lot about disproportion. The discovery of acids and their properties could fit in very well with the old Hippocratic tradition. The new science indicated that acid substances were a normal constituent of the body. Sylvius made a great advance by indicating that acid, if disproportionate in amount or quality, could produce disease. And the use of alkalis to counteract the acid was completely logical. We cannot condemn Sylvius for his ignorance of bacteria, any more than we can condemn today's physicians for not knowing the results of tomorrow's researches.

Sylvius, as a leading physician of his era, drew upon contemporary science to explain the phenomena of health and disease. He used the science of his time to build a conceptual framework for medicine, and at the same time he tried to harmonize the new views with traditional attitudes. To be sure, his doctrines were wrong, but in the history of science this is a minor detail.

Let me present another example drawn from anatomy rather than from chemistry. In the late seventeenth century Frederick Ruysch, a prominent Dutch anatomist, perfected new technical methods of vascular injection, whereby he was able to demonstrate with remarkable clarity the vascular pattern in different organs. His new technique showed the enormous complexity of the vasculature, and the different vascular patterns that characterize different parts of the body. As is so often the case when a new technique provides new experimental data, Ruysch's findings gave great impetus to medical science, analogous, perhaps, to that which electron microscopy has furnished in the past thirty years.

New data, the fruit of advancing technology, can modify the basic concepts in a science. And yet, when new concepts arise, physicians try to harmonize the recent information with existing knowledge and traditional concepts. Ruysch's discoveries had a substantial effect on medical theory. The great Hermann Boerhaave (1668–1738), the most prominent physician in the first half of the eighteenth century, adapted the data of vascular injection to elaborate some new explanatory principles.

In the eighteenth century various humors were well recognized—saliva, bile, milk, pancreatic juice, sweat, tears, mucus, urine—all these derived from the blood, and all of them had their own characteristic properties. The liver did not secrete milk, nor the kidneys saliva, nor the pancreas bile. How did the specificity come about? Today we can glibly call on cell theory, but in the eighteenth century this was unknown. Yet the very existence of specific secretions cried out for an explanation. The ancients had offered the concept of "faculties"—the breast, they would have said, had a milk-producing faculty. The eighteenth century, however, called for a different concept, derived from more contemporary science.

Wanting to utilize the current scientific advances, Boerhaave correlated the observed differences among the secretions with the observed differences in blood vessels.[7] The secretions all came ultimately from the blood, and the blood passed through various glands. The glands, therefore, must differ somehow one from the other. How? The new science indicated that in the various glands the blood-vessel patterns varied greatly one from the other. To account for specificity, Boerhaave invoked such factors as the distance of the arteries from the heart, the angle an artery made with the parent stem, the pattern of the arterioles, the number of ramifications, the velocity of the blood, the degree of stasis. Thus, he said, "the small arteriolae of the pituitary membrane are strait, in the spleen they form penicilli or bunches like pencil brushes, in the kidneys they take a serpentine or vermicular course, in the lungs and elsewhere they form plexuses or networks . . ."[8] These anatomical variations, he thought, would affect the course of the blood, which would be now slower, now more rapid; would strike the sides with greater or less force; or would be more or less compacted, according to the configuration of the vessels. *These factors, he thought, helped to sort out the different materials in the bloodstream.* This attempt to explain the specificity of secretions is far from despicable. It so happens that Boerhaave was wrong, but such a fate sooner or later overtakes all scientists.

An obvious criticism comes to mind. Boerhaave and Sylvius, according to our standards, had little basis for their assertions. A bit of initial evidence there was, but not anything that we would regard as cogent. Sylvius could point to a few unquestionable facts, for example, that strong acids applied to the skin would produce an inflammation and even cause an ulceration. But on this slender basis Sylvius engaged in a chain of inference, ending with the claim that inflammation and ulceration could come from acids *inside* the body, from acids in the bloodstream. And for this he had no *direct* sup-

[7] Lester S. King, *Medical World of the Eighteenth Century* (Chicago: University of Chicago Press, 1958), chaps. 3 and 4 passim.

[8] Hermann Boerhaave, *Academical Lectures on the Theory of Physic*, 6 vols. (London, 1741–1757, first and second editions intermingled), 2 (1743), 235.

portive evidence. Similarly, Boerhaave could point to sound experimental data that different organs or glands had different vascular patterns. No one could deny it. But then he inferred that these differences were somehow responsible for the specific secretions, and for this inference he had no direct evidence.

Both Sylvius and Boerhaave started with facts, upon which they superimposed various assumptions and inferences. Today we might call it pure speculation, but this, I feel, is an improper evaluation. The doctrines were based on initial evidence, together with inferential elaboration. We would say that there was but a miniscule amount of evidence and a vast quantity of inference, and, far more important, there was no added supportive evidence for the asserted conclusions.

This criticism is unquestionably true, but it omits the crucial feature—that *these men did not see the need for supportive evidence.* Sylvius and Boerhaave were keen observers, well versed in their contemporary science; they studied nature and tried to explain the causes operative in medicine. Reasoning carefully, they used the scientific concepts of their day to explain the phenomena of disease. They believed that they were properly scientific. Their concept of scientific medicine, unlike that of today, did not involve the need for supportive evidence. They were laboring in a different cultural environment.

In the cultural environment of the seventeenth and eighteenth centuries, belief flourished on scanty initial evidence. One single observation might supply the groundwork for a great deal of logical elaboration. Physicians might take a few concrete data and immediately expand them into broad general principles, in the same way that some candy vendors can take a small amount of sugar and blow it up into a great froth of spun sugar candy.

The real development of scientific medicine—what perhaps we so chauvinistically call "modern" medicine—involved a change in attitude rather than merely a series of new discoveries. If I were asked to identify the cornerstone of medical science, I would point to two connected concepts—first, the realization that logical coherence is not enough to establish a claim, but that empirical evidence is necessary. And second, the evidence must be evaluated, and critical evaluation must be applied to both empirical data and derived theories. *The critical attitude, and not any particular discovery, is the real core of scientific medicine.* Historians can trace the slow, painful growth of critical attitude and note its relationship with cultural factors.

Scientific medicine I equate with the search for validity, the appreciation of controls, the need for checking and rechecking, the search for negative instances and alternative explanations. Many seventeenth-century medical investigators showed these qualities to an admirable degree, but most medical practitioners did not. There was all too great a readiness to jump to conclusions, to assert general principles on the basis of scanty data. This tendency characterized the general cultural stream, despite such occasional brilliant exceptions as William Harvey.

However, a slow cultural transformation occurred in the seventeenth, eighteenth, and nineteenth centuries, with a renewed emphasis on observation and cautious inference, and a less hasty jumping to conclusions. A new empiricism developed, with Francis Bacon as its great seventeenth-century representative, and John Stuart Mill, Auguste Comte, Karl Pearson, and Henri Poincaré as some of its nineteenth-century exemplars. Medicine shared in this transformation and I wish to give briefly two different examples.

The first goes back to the eighteenth century. At that time scurvy, which is virtually wiped out today, was a widespread and dreaded disease. It would almost always attack men who were on ships that remained far from land for a prolonged period of time. Its nature was unknown and there was not even any definite way of making a clear-cut diagnosis. Many symptoms were rather constant, such as bleeding, spongy gums, hemorrhages, and prostration, but the clinical picture was complicated and various other symptoms were sometimes considered important, sometimes not. These included vomiting and diarrhea, ulcerations, skin changes, edema, mental changes. Often physicians could not agree on which patients actually had scurvy; one physician might make the diagnosis and another might deny it. There were no generally accepted remedies, just as there was no generally accepted theory of etiology.

James Lind, an eighteenth-century Scottish naval surgeon, performed a brilliant clinical study to discover the basic nature of scurvy.[9] Born in 1716, Lind had an apprenticeship in medicine and then became a naval surgeon. In 1753 he published a monumental book on scurvy that unfortunately attracted all too little attention, but nevertheless stands as a model of scientific medicine.

To determine how scurvy might be prevented and cured, Lind carried out a fine experiment. During one of his voyages, when scurvy was rife, he took twelve severely ill patients, as similar as he could pick. He kept them all on a uniform diet. Dividing the patients into six groups of two men each, he gave each group a specific medication in addition to their basic diet. For example, one pair received a quart of cider a day; another, an elixir of vitriol (a form of sulfuric acid) and a gargle; another, sea water; another, vinegar. To one pair he gave citrus fruit, two oranges and a lemon each day. Unfortunately, there was only enough fruit to last them six days.

The results of this experiment were dramatic and clear-cut. The men who ate the oranges and lemons showed extraordinary improvement. One of the pair recovered to such a degree that he could go back to active duty. The other did not do quite so well but made sufficient progress to enable him to nurse the other patients. Of the ten remaining men, the two who drank the cider did better than the others, but far less well than did those who ate the citrus fruit.

The data seemed quite unequivocal and the conclusions clear-cut, but Lind was not satisfied and tried to find possible errors. For example, lemons and oranges contain acid. Perhaps, he thought, it might be the acid component in the citrus fruit that had the healing power. To eliminate this possible objection he pointed to vinegar and to elixir of vitriol, both of which were acids. These, although commonly used on shipboard, neither prevented nor cured scurvy. Hence, acid as such was not the important factor.

[9] *Lind's Treatise on Scurvy*, a reprint of the first edition of *A Treatise on Scurvy* (1753), ed. C. P. Stewart and D. Guthrie (Edinburgh: University Press, 1953).

The actual curative agent he did not identify. The concept of vitamins was not defined until the twentieth century, but this lack of identification does not in any way detract from the excellence of Lind's experiments nor from the clarity of his thought. He did not have complicated apparatus but he did have critical judgment and the ability to evaluate evidence, and he recognized the need for controls and for criteria which could distinguish a chance association from a real causal effect. He had the clear insight that some evidence was good, other evidence not good; that some evidence could give rise to valid and reliable conclusions, while from poor evidence no conclusions could emerge. In addition, he realized that conclusions and generalizations must have a solid foundation and should not soar off into flimsy imaginings. He tried to examine the facts objectively. Lind was a fine example of the medical scientist who attended to experience and did so with critical judgment. He made rational inferences, but his inferences had at all times a close relationship to concrete experience.

There is an unhappy irony in this account. Despite Lind's convincing demonstration regarding the role of citrus fruit in curing scurvy, his ideas did not find ready acceptance until much later. It was not enough for a few individuals to have a clear perception of validity and a sound evaluation of evidence. Such an attitude had to become part of the whole cultural pattern, and the mid-eighteenth century was still struggling to throw off the old pattern.

Now let us jump some seventy-five years or so into the nineteenth century and regard the practice of bloodletting. This procedure was, for over two thousand years, a mainstay of therapeutics, a major weapon wherewith physicians tried to repel disease. The evidence that supported bloodletting was quite simple and direct: the patient was sick; the doctor let blood; the patient recovered. This, of course, represents the so-called *post hoc ergo propter hoc* reasoning that draws a causal relationship on the basis of temporal relationship. The value of bloodletting also received support from theoretical considerations. *Why* bloodletting was effective the physician could always explain by referring to various humors and the circulation, to congestion and stasis and hydrodynamic principles. Most of the great physicians of the seventeenth and eighteenth centuries believed in bloodletting and justified their belief by pointing to concrete experience on the one hand—the patients got well—and to logical theories on the other.

Even if physicians had quite opposing theories *why* bloodletting helped, they nevertheless would agree that it *did* help. The uncritical acceptance of alleged facts and the reliance on theory to justify the acceptance reflected the general cultural attitude that was common in the eighteenth century.

In the nineteenth century, however, the new empiricism became more widespread, with important consequences. The younger physicians, especially those in France who had grown up in the Napoleonic era, showed a far greater skepticism toward theory and a much greater concern with facts. Such men as Bayle, Laennec, Louis, Bretonneau, and Chomel were much more empirically minded than their predecessors. They were far more critical regarding what they would accept as fact and what inferences might be derived therefrom.

One of the leaders in this group, Pierre C. A. Louis, was quite dissatisfied with the evidence on which rested the alleged value of bloodletting. He reexamined the evidence and, by exerting appropriate controls, tried to test the effectiveness of bloodletting. His conclusions, actually, were largely erroneous, but his critical attitude was magnificent. We can see how crude was his method and how hampered he was by inadequate concepts of disease and of statistics. But these are minor details. For all his errors, he provided a mighty impetus to the development of scientific medicine, and his so-called numerical method introduced quantitative method into clinical studies.

Louis studied the effects of bloodletting on various diseases.[10] For our purposes his observations on pneumonia are particularly important. He carried out a retrospective study, that is, he examined the

[10] P. C. A. Louis, *Researches on the Effects of Blood-letting in Some Inflammatory Diseases*, trans. C. G. Putnam (Boston: Hillard Gray and Co., 1836).

records of cases and, noting various factors, tried to find out what effect bloodletting had had on the progress and termination of the disease. He considered different variables. Some of the factors that he took into account were the duration of the disease, the number of bloodlettings, the stage of the disease when the bloodletting occurred, the patient's age, other therapy, and symptoms.

He prepared certain tables that would facilitate the comparison of data, and he drew certain cautious conclusions. He was able to show that, when the records were critically examined, the alleged benefit derived from bloodletting was far less than was generally supposed. On the positive side, he concluded that bloodletting, if carried out in the first four days of the disease, had a favorable effect—the patients recovered four or five days sooner than those bled at a later period. He considered, further, that the age of the patient exerted great influence on the progress and outcome of the disease, and inferred that bloodletting, carried out in the early stages, never arrests the disease all at once.

As for other remedies, he believed that blistering—another favorite and time-honored remedy—was entirely without effect. But in severe cases, where bloodletting had proved ineffective, antimony in large doses appeared to diminish the mortality.

Louis's importance in medical history does not rest on any concrete discoveries, for he did not make any significant discoveries. But he is important for the cautious analytical attitude that he adopted; his respect for facts; his insistence on the actual enumeration of instances and quantitative comparison of data; the need for controls; and above all for the way in which he influenced a whole generation of young physicians and inspired them to embrace the new empiricism. Compared with these merits, the defects in his methods are of little importance.

The new empiricism did not neglect the scientist's duty to provide explanations. It did not abandon theory, but it did introduce new standards of evaluation. It strengthened the critical attitude and thereby emphasized the difficulties of scientific endeavor.

Scientific medicine, whether clinical or experimental, has always had the twin tasks of finding the data and then explaining the data.

But the explanation, to qualify as scientific, must be good. It must withstand critical analysis. The critical physician constantly asks himself such questions as, Is it true? How do I know? Have I adequate controls? What are the alternatives? These questions reflect an attitude of mind, an attitude which, to become widespread, must form a part of the whole pervading culture. While in the past 150 years the concepts of scientific rigor have penetrated more and more into the cultural milieu, they still have reached only a small percentage of physicians.

Scientific medicine does not depend on gadgets or tests, or on sharply precise results; neither does it imply the capacity to cure the patient. It does require the ability to examine the data, to seek the connections between them, to find an explanation, and in all these processes, to apply critical acumen.

Ethical Problems of Medical Research

HENRY K. BEECHER, M.D.
Harvard University Medical School

The Stage

As one wanders around the white marble quadrangle of the Harvard Medical School, a bizarre idea is thrust at him, sometimes loud and clear, sometimes muted, but always insistently there. It is the view that the true scientist studies only electrons and ions, atoms and molecules, the frog and the dog, that any time he concerns himself directly with mankind he has strayed—regrettably—far downstream from heaven.

Along with everybody else I am bored with arguments of basic vs. applied science. The basic scientist discovers and establishes new concepts, all else is applied science, whether it be in a laboratory of physics or at the bedside of a sick man. I once, brashly, arranged a series of twenty Lowell Lectures to illustrate this theme; four of the essayists—Nobel laureates Pauling, Richards, Cori, Enders—described how the significant advances they had made originated at the bedside of a sick man.

The university hospitals of the land have long been recognized as fields where concepts already discovered are applied, but now it is evident that they are the *only* places where certain discoveries basic to the advancement of pure science are likely to occur. Such institutions are indispensable units in the advancement of some aspects of conceptual science. In short, a new role of the great teaching hospital is emerging: the advancement of conceptual science through studies of man.

This awareness leads to a further extension of human experimentation: having seen what fundamental ends can be achieved by experimentation in man, the investigator is led to carry on where Nature leaves off. His purposes thus become deeper and more complex than ever before and so also do the ethical problems surrounding them. Anything to do with experimentation in man has relevance to both basic and applied science.

I intend to concentrate on one small area: the interface between the investigator and his human subject. For some years now a host of important issues has been stated, challenged, argued, debated, fought over, agreed upon, defended, until I sometimes believe I am caught up in a Kafka nightmare. There seems to be endless reiteration of the truth, but nothing new. I am not denigrating the importance of, for example, the definition of experimentation in man; justification for the human trial; the frequency of unethical or questionably ethical practices; valid consent and the engineering of consent; volunteers and their frequent psychopathology; the perils of using captive groups as subjects, whether ward patients, children, students, prisoners, or the dying; the doctor-patient relationship vs. the doctor-subject relationship; the ethical problems arising in the transplant of tissues and organs; the Kefauver-Harris Amendments, the FDA, and their effects on experimentation and medical progress; the definition of death—and so on and on.

These problems are, to be sure, important, and nearly everybody has had his say about them—to the extent that it is unlikely anything *fresh* can soon be said about them. But I believe there is another group of less obvious, relatively little discussed, but equally important problems relevant to experimentation in man, and I would like to take a look at them.

These inadequately faced areas are inseparable from the tight little microcosm of the investigator and his subject—for example, self-experimentation (when the investigator is also his subject!); invasion of privacy; deception; trust; "statistical" morality; ends, means, and morals; situation ethics; and the individual vs. society.

The investigator and his subject do not exist, as the cliché has it, in a vacuum, so I shall have to make brief reference to some of the situations that surround them. The much debated informed or valid consent is such a one. In all but the simplest situations this is only a goal toward which we strive, but strive we must for legal, social, and moral reasons. Often the goal is quite unreachable in any truly satisfactory sense, but in our striving the subject at least becomes aware that he is to *be* the subject of an experiment and can refuse to participate if he chooses to do so. I have discussed elsewhere the too often confused myths and realities of consent (5).

I have deliberately plunged into the midst of the difficult problems of experimentation in man. The recent furor in this area might lead a young man to believe that these matters were newly arisen.

A Historical Note on Self-Experimentation

The oldest world literatures contain references to experimental work with both animals and man. It was the practice in ancient Persia for the king to hand over condemned criminals for experimental purposes in science. The Ptolemies used criminals in Egypt, and so did Fallopius in Pisa during the Renaissance. "A Persian prince at the time of Avicenna was giving advice to a young man who was going to join the medical profession. He said, 'Once you embark on a career as a physician if you wish to gain experience and a reputation you must experiment freely, but you had better not choose people of high rank or political importance for your subjects' " (25).

While human experimentation has accompanied the practice of medicine from times of antiquity, the current concept of planned medical research has not really been presented as such to the courts. As the courts have understood it, human experimentation has not been, nor is it now, *legally* recognized as a legitimate part of the physician's activities except as this may be necessary in treating a patient, with his consent, or in preparing for his treatment as required by the Food and Drug Administration's drug-testing program. Even so, any slips and the investigator is threatened with a brush with the law where precedent says that a man experiments to his peril. The universal and long-standing recognition that human research is essential to the advancement of medical science and the newer recognition that some aspects of even basic science cannot advance without it have led to a correct, although still in most cases extra-legal, expansion of human experimentation. Curiously, such work, when well conceived and soundly conducted, is everywhere recognized as being properly within the ethical and moral concepts of our time; but it is not yet broadly recognized in law.

Experimentation on other men requires a *willingness* to experiment upon oneself as evidence of good faith, although in a given case self-experimentation may be wholly impractical. When it is carried out, it must be done with the same safeguards that are applied to other subjects. Ivy (16) cites a number of examples to indicate that willingness without the discipline of proper controls can be misleading, or devastating, or both, to the self-experimenting participant: There was the case of John Hunter who inoculated himself, in 1767, with gonorrheal pus to prove the disease transmissible in this way. He succeeded. But from the same inoculum he also acquired syphilis, and concluded that gonorrhea and syphilis were merely manifestations of the same disease. Purkinjé gave himself enough digitalis to kill nine cats in order to study its effects on his own vision. He had cardiac pain and irregularity and vomited for a week. Hales, enthusiastic about the marvels of intravenous injection, received a half ounce of castor oil by this route and lived to describe its remarkable effects. Tonery, in 1830, in order to convince the French Academy of the extraordinary powers of charcoal to absorb alkaloids, took, with this safeguard, a dose of strychnine which would have been lethal without it. In 1857, carbon tetrachloride was tried out as an anesthetic in man; a few animal experiments would have shown it to be unsuitable. In 1894 Oliver told Professor Schafer that he had made extracts of all of the endocrine glands and injected them into his own son. Schafer altered the experiment and was the first to demonstrate the pressor effect of epinephrine in dogs and cats. Ivy concludes that "these experiments may be a tribute to the enthusiasm and bravery of these early medical scientists, but they clearly show the limitations and dangers of uncontrolled self-experimentation."

The Invasion of Privacy

But now to come to some of the subtleties that impinge on the microcosm of the investigator and his subject, that is, the invasion of privacy.

As ancient as the common law is the principle that the individual shall be protected in his person and in his property. Starting from this, Warren and Brandeis (30) long ago recognized that "political, social and economic changes entail the recognition of new rights, and the common law, in its eternal youth, grows to meet the demands of society. . . . Later there came a recognition of man's spiritual nature, of his feelings and his intellect. Gradually the scope of these legal rights broadened; and now the right to life has come to mean the right to enjoy life,—the right to be let alone." Thus, nearly eighty years ago there was recognition by legal scholars of the value of sensations, "feelings," enjoyment, recognition that a man had a right to his privacy, privacy so often and so casually threatened in experimentation.

There is indeed an aspect of the investigator's activities which has had too little attention up to the present—his sometimes offhand invasion of the privacy of his subject. All signs indicate that the matter is to be widely examined in the immediate future. This area is of such importance in human experimentation that it requires a rather extensive presentation. As a basic principle, intrusion into a human body or mind under any and all circumstances is no more permissible than casual search and seizure in a house.

On looking backward for a moment, it is evident that the modern origins of an interest in privacy stem from the historic study of the subject by Mr. Warren and the young Brandeis. This was published in 1890, after some years of work. The word *privacy* thus appeared in legal literature for the first time. (In the United States Constitution nothing is said about privacy.)

Ernst and Schwartz (13) refer to the Warren and Brandeis study as "a spurt of legal imagination which takes us far beyond what at the time were considered by many to be immutable principles of law and logic. Here are Warren and Brandeis in 1890, ambushing from the previous . . . cases the perhaps unspoken elements that bound them all together at that time, and moulding these elements into a new legal principle that deftly expresses what all the inadequate fumblings of the past had not been able or inclined to do."

Sometimes epoch-making events have their origins in trivial situations, and that was the case here: the Warrens were active in the Back Bay social life of the late nineteenth century. It was their custom to give frequent dinner parties, and there was a great scrambling by the press to find out who would be present. The attempted invasion of his privacy annoyed Warren and was the passing occasion for his persistent interest in the matter. He sought the collaboration of the young Brandeis, and American Law has not been the same since.

The invasion of privacy by the investigator takes many forms, among them the countless questionnaires with their sometimes impertinent questions, beginning at the grade-school level and continuing through job applications, married life, and on into senescence. Those who are supported by public welfare funds can expect official invasion of their privacy; so also can the entire population during data gathering for the government's census. Even though the original aims of such studies may be correct, there is always the danger that the accumulated data may eventually be used for unintended purposes. Jury rooms have been bugged, with the cooperation not only of the courts but also of the most august organizations. (28). Mankind is spied on, recorded, reported on, and harassed by a gamut of devices and persons ranging from the simpleminded Peeping Tom to the devilishly complex and effective electronic surveillance techniques. Some of this spying is motivated by competition in business or by domestic tangles, some of it is for criminal purposes, some of it is for law enforcement, but much of it is for "research"; hence comment is appropriate in the present considerations.

When the collection of data is mandatory, as in certain governmental procedures, in industry, or in welfare situations, there is a great burden on the sponsoring agency to protect the subject against disclosure unless disclosure is specifically arranged for by the individuals concerned or by statute. There are sometimes regulations to be observed, as in the case of the physician who is required by law to report venereal disease.

While only a small proportion of the population may be exposed to serious invasions of privacy, as the report of the panel on privacy and behavioral research points out (26), there is enough of such action against the minority to "risk eroding the quality of life for the majority."

The extent of the invasion of privacy can hardly be surprising to those familiar with behavioral research, for the social sciences, political science, economics, anthropology, sociology, and psychology are all concerned with the behavior of individuals, of groups, of communities. In 1966 some 35,000 behavioral scientists were engaged in such research in the United States; 2,100 new Ph.D.'s pour forth each year; 40,000 students are presently seeking advanced degrees in the behavioral sciences. In 1966 the federal government contributed 300 million dollars to behavioral research (26).

The individual's right to be let alone conflicts with the advancement of society based upon scientific research, where the purposes of behavioral studies are concerned with the assessment and measurement of many qualities of man's mind, feelings, and actions. There is, clearly, conflict between the individual's right to seclusion and, in many areas, the right of the public to be informed. So also is there conflict between the role of privacy and the guarantee of free speech and a free press. The violation of privacy is an indignity to the individual. The concern for privacy arises in concern for the individual. In a totalitarian state only the dictator is allowed privacy.

When studies are made without the consent of the subject they constitute an invasion of privacy that can be serious; but at the same time it must be recognized that prior discussion of the work planned can distort the results; thus the honest investigator has a dilemma not easily resolved. In the end, most scientists in the field accept something short of the ideal; a situation where a state of mutual trust exists between scientist and subject, where the latter's dignity and anonymity are preserved.

In his inquiry into the autonomy of the individual, Shils (28) recognized that respect for privacy is a rather recent addition to the values of modern liberalism, that the value of privacy is derived from our belief in "the sacredness of individuality." This must be respected by the investigator. Deception is contrary to such respect. Privacy can be suspended only by the deliberate decision of the subject involved, except, as I say, where sanctioned by statute as in the required reporting of venereal disease.

The panel on privacy (26) concluded that "neither the principle of privacy nor the need to discover new knowledge can supervene universally." As with other conflicts in our society, according to the panel there is need for adjustment and compromise in determining which value is to govern a given situation. The cost in privacy is balanced against the gain in knowledge, leaving one with a feeling of uneasiness—a fear that the individual will be sacrificed, as illustrated by the following quotation from the same report: "Furthermore, the investigator is first and foremost a scientist in search of new knowledge, and it would not be in accord with our understanding of human motivation to expect him always to be as vigilant for his subject's welfare as he is for the productiveness of his own research."

Nor is it reassuring to find the panel concluding, "If intrusion on privacy proves essential to the research, he [the investigator] should not proceed with his proposed experiment until he and his colleagues have considered all of the relevant facts and he has determined, with support from them, that the benefits outweigh the costs." Unfortunately, one must say it again: Ends may not justify means. Unfortunately also, in the report's concluding remarks there does not seem to be any awareness that some experiments simply cannot be carried out—science is not always the highest good.

Complex as is the individual's right to a private personality, this is not nearly as secure in law as the right to private property, as Ruebhausen and Brim (18) point out. There are, nonetheless, two major aspects of it: there is the "right to be let alone," so movingly attested to by Judge Cooley (10), and there is "the right to share and to communicate" (18).

While the individual strives always to protect his privacy, the collection of individuals and institutions called "society" tends always to invade it. Serious or not, the important test is this: Is the threat or the invasion by the investigator unreasonable or intolerable (18)?

These instruments and techniques have been developed in response to the operational methods employed by organized criminals. It must be admitted that the instruments have created unique problems for law enforcement officers as well as for scientific investigators. It would be fair to ask: Who has the right to overhear, and for what purpose? And if such eavesdropping is permitted, how is it to be limited or controlled? Hubert Humphrey has written (*Life*, April 2, 1967), "We act differently if we believe we are being observed. If we can never be sure whether or not we are being watched and listened to, all our actions will be altered and our very character will change." Justice Brennan, in the same issue, spoke of another aspect of this dark subject: "Electronic aids add a wholly new dimension to eavesdropping. They make it more penetrating, more indiscriminate, more truly obnoxious to a free society. Electronic surveillance, in fact, makes the police omniscient; and police omniscience is one of the most effective tools of tyranny."

The Threat to Privacy: Bugging

One dare not overlook the threat to privacy inherent in the field of electronic surveillance. Privacy of communication is essential among citizens. Fear or suspicion that one's activities in speech are being supervised by a stranger has a seriously inhibiting effect upon a willingness to present critical and constructive ideas. "When dissent from the popular view is discouraged, intellectual controversy is smothered, the process for testing new concepts and ideas is hindered and desirable change is slowed. External restraints, of which electronic surveillance is but one possibility, are thus repugnant to citizens of such a society" (11, p. 202).

The development of electronic surveillance techniques in recent years has been remarkable; the electronic cocktail olive is only one illustration. Parabolic microphones can pick up conversations held in the open hundreds of feet away. These microphones can be purchased commercially. Laser beams have shown promise in picking up conversations within a room by focusing on a windowpane. Further progress has led to the production of equipment of extremely small size. Bugging can detect and provide for a record of what is said anywhere. It is not dependent upon the telephone; it seriously threatens privacy.

Just how widespread such surveillance activities really are is not known. Many who employ these techniques are fearful that their conduct may be declared unlawful and thus are not willing to report their activities. This applies to scientific investigators as well as to others. Individuals familiar with the field believe that electronic surveillance is widely present and its use rapidly increasing. The threat to privacy is very great indeed. We have entered the electronic age, with its appalling possibilities for the invasion of privacy. It is all too easy to rationalize this as being required by science.

The tools just mentioned facilitate the scientific invasion of privacy; but one must not lose sight of the fact that a serious invasion of privacy is the use of subjects in experimentation without their knowledge or specific consent.

Other Types of Invasion of Privacy

Modell (23) makes the point that in earlier years when drugs were evaluated empirically, the disasters that followed this method were not very apparent, but now, with carefully planned evaluation of drugs, great attention is being drawn to the medical scientist's activities, with the result that he is sometimes "pilloried for his meticulousness." The over-all result is that the medical scientist is wrongfully placed on the defensive.

Modern sciences and technologies have given rise to major health hazards which lead to an invasion of the private person without his knowledge or consent, but, like medicine in an earlier year, since no attempt was made to estimate the hazard, these sciences and technologies have remained free to expose masses of people in an unlimited way. As examples Modell cites the contamination of the air, the soil, the watersheds, and the water by industrial wastes. Such contamination has only recently become a matter of organized concern, applied especially to automobile exhausts in the air and detergents in the soil. No careful experiments have been carried out to determine the extent of these hazards and therefore they have not yet been labeled "inhumane."

Inconsistencies abound in degrees of regulation. "The Food and Drug Administration does not require the application of any of the ethical safeguards for human subjects exposed to insecticides in experiments that it requires for medicinal drugs, even though the former are by their very nature toxic. The Government participated with the airplane industry in an experiment to determine the effects on mind and body of repeated frequent sonic booms involving all the inhabitants of Oklahoma City without anyone's permission. And, of course, we are all subjects of a still unfinished long-term chronic experiment on the effects of ionization to which no one willingly or knowingly gave consent" (12). Experimentation without consent is not uncommon in government circles. In this same context Cahn (8) has said, "I wish to suggest that, in the areas of scientific interest which impinge on government and law, there are limits to the permissibility of experimentation, that the limits are imposed by institutional factors on one hand and moral factors on the other, and that they require much more attention and respect than lawyers, ethicists, or experimental scientists have been giving them." It would seem only reasonable that the same ethical consideration should apply to all controllable exposures, not to the medical alone. "We are obligated to discover the size of the hazard by preliminary trial or experiment in man; and . . . a meaningful ethical basis for their operation will be developed only when all the influences of scientific and technologic progress on man's health are, as with drugs, examined in disciplined experiments before mass exposure. This is the primary ethical decision" (8).

When diagnosis or therapy for the benefit of the given individual is at stake, such invasion of his privacy or his body can be proper, for the individual has, in the act of coming to the physician for relief, already given consent to reasonable efforts to relieve him. But when such invasion takes place without the knowledge or consent of the individual involved, and not for his benefit, it evokes, when exposed, a powerful and hostile public reaction, however well motivated the perpetrators considered themselves to be. Physical transgressions are easy enough to find and to identify. The subtle invasions of the private personality are more difficult to single out. The public reaction against such acts has been and is likely to be violent, and this violence inevitably leads to harsh and arbitrary restrictions.

It would be most unfortunate if the social scientist became identified in the public mind with violations of privacy, with snooping. It is unthinkable to accept progress in medicine founded on deceit, on a subject defrauded of his privacy or his physical safety. Such methods run counter to almost all that medicine stands for.

Deception by the Investigator in Human Experimentation

Deception in human experimentation can take various forms, some of which are legitimate, if hedged about with certain restrictions and requirements, some of which are not legitimate. Worst of all is the risk of patients' health or life without their knowledge and consent. It will be helpful to take a look at the several kinds of deception.

Placebos. These provide good examples of the point just made—some deception is defensible and some is not. First, the defensible: when a patient comes to a doctor for relief, he gives, in the act of coming, his consent to reasonable efforts to relieve him. The physician may very properly wish to pit a drug the patient has been receiving against a placebo, to see if the drug has any specific value. This is in the patient's interest. The information cannot be obtained in any other way and the temporary deceit is acceptable.

Another example: A placebo is not "nothing." It is a powerful therapeutic tool (2, 17) with, on the average, about one-half to two-thirds the power of morphine in the usual dose in relieving severe pain. In the presence of stress, under special circumstances, the placebo may have more than three-quarters the effectiveness of morphine in relieving pain (3, 4). There is no requirement that the physician always use the most powerful therapeutic agent in treatment. The more powerful the agent is, the more powerful its accompanying undesirable side effects will usually be. Thus the deception inherent in the use of a placebo in some therapeutic situations can be legitimate.

The above examples emerge from therapy. When placebos are used in experimental work with volunteers, the situation changes. Some will argue that if no discernible risk is involved, the secret use of placebos is legitimate—if disclosure of their presence would vitiate the information sought. The argument is a dubious one at best. In most cases, if not in all, a statement to the volunteers that they *may* get a placebo suffices; but it must be explained to them that they will not know if or when this will be. The subjects thus have the right to accept or reject the situation. If they accept it, the deception they will experience is legitimate. This of course applies to other kinds of deception as well as to placebos.

"*Stooges.*" Instead of the unpleasant term "deception," the more felicitous but tricky term, "unannounced observations," is sometimes used. However it is put, an unfavorable picture emerges. One wonders why so little is said about it in the President's panel on privacy and behavioral research (26). Without approving or disapproving comment the panel seems to accept the existence of deception in research and thereby gives approval of a sort. One study is mentioned in which all subjects present in a room are stooges, except one. The point of interest is how the judgment of that one may be affected by the deliberately misleading influence of the stooges. Following the deception, the subject is told the purpose of the study and its results. An experiment of this sort may put a subject under stress and raise self-doubts.

Margaret Mead (20), with characteristic eloquence and forthrightness, has taken sharp issue with the use of stooges:

> Is it scientifically and ethically permissible to deceive the subjects of research by disguising oneself as a "participant observer," or by introducing stooges into an experiment, or by making use of long-distance television or hidden microphones or other devices for concealed observation? When a human being is introduced who is consciously distorting

his position, the material of the research is inevitably jeopardized, and the results always are put in question as the "participant"—introduced as a "psychotic" into a mental ward or as a "fanatic" into a flying-saucer cult group—gives his subjects false clues of a non-verbal nature and produces distortions which cannot be traced in his results. Concealed instruments of observation may not distort the subjects' course of action, but the subsequent revelation of their presence—as in the jury room that was tapped for sociological purposes—damages the trust both of the original participants and of all others who come to know about it. The deception violates the conventions of privacy and human dignity and casts scientists in the role of spies, intelligence agents, Peeping Toms, and versions of Big Brother. Furthermore, it damages science by cutting short attempts to construct methods of research that would responsibly enhance, rather than destroy, human trust.

In a further discussion of this problem several years later, Margaret Mead (21) points out that the "primary consideration is whether the human beings who are involved shall either be lied to or asked to lie to others, i.e., to function as stooges." Her arguments can be summarized: If one fails to acquaint the experimental subject with what is happening, within reasonable limits, one reduces his stature as a human being in that he has not been permitted to judge for himself. All problems are not solved by "debriefing" the man. He is told he has been tricked, deluded, spied upon, and lied to. Acceptance of such information requires that the subject identify himself with the lying investigator or reach "the decision that social science is a bunch of confidence tricks and now he also knows a few" (21). If the subject cannot use such self-satisfying rationalizations he can consider himself abused. Or he may decide that being lied to is merely the price he must pay for some other advantage sought—education, preferment, and so on. And all of this can lead to a cynical attitude toward such experimentation.

Deceit can, in some situations, have a more serious effect on the investigator than on the deceived subject. The tricky investigator becomes accustomed to deceiving and manipulating other human beings. Even though this is explained after the fact to the subject, it still carries the implication that the manipulation of people is acceptable. Contempt for others grows out of this. The investigator becomes omnipotent. This is a threat to the integrity of his own scientific work.

It must be acknowledged that deceit may be necessary and if, as mentioned earlier, the subject is aware of this possibility and accepts it, even though he is temporarily demeaned as a human being, it must sometimes be accepted. For example, the fabricated situations and the use of stooges to test the strength and resilience of astronauts comes to mind, also the means of selecting candidates for dangerous secret activities in warfare or in exploration. Even here, the important question is whether the deception is absolutely necessary in an experiment which is itself required.

As for the effect of deception on the experiment, the first question is, Does the experimental design absolutely require deception of the subject? Next, Is an experiment which incorporates deception ever a *valid* experiment? (21). One must accept the well-demonstrated fact that many individuals are able to pick up cues that others are not aware of giving, and one or more of the subjects may realize that the investigator is lying. This is impossible to control and the validity of the experiment is jeopardized thereby. It may be possible to get around the unconscious delivery of cues by the use of mechanical guides or mechanical instructors, which, if cleverly and imaginatively arranged, will spare the subject the feeling of being deceived by the experimenter. "If the potential invalidity of all experiments where lying occurs is recognized, this will stimulate the use of other kinds of experiments" (21).

Trust

As science becomes more and more significant in the modern world, it is absolutely essential that this be a *trusted* activity. "The image of the scientist as someone who is trustworthy and humane is impaired every time that there are accounts of research which have disregarded basic human rights of consent, as in revelations about medical experiments on unconsenting patients, or scientists using lying, deceit, disguises and spying in the collection of data, or misquoting or suppressing evidence in the discussion of public policy.

. . . Trust in the responsible use of power is essential for an ordered society. Trust in the responsible use of knowledge, which increasingly gives overweaning power, is crucial today" (21).

Margaret Mead's opening comment at the 1968 American Academy of Arts and Sciences Conference on Human Experimentation (22) epitomizes the requirement for most such work. She said that although her field of anthropological research does not have subjects, "*We work with informants in an atmosphere of trust and mutual respect*" (italics mine). This is as broad as the Golden Rule; it is the basic requirement for ethical experimentation in man. I should like to refer to several more of her points in the material immediately following.

It is the scientist's responsibility to the subjects that they not be exposed to ridicule, or legal sanctions, or danger (without their informed concurrence). Thoughtless invasion of privacy is not to be tolerated. The trustworthy investigator will not overlook his obligation to his own discipline as well as to the public image of scientific work. "The more powerless the subject is, per se, the more the question of ethics—and power—is raised . . . It is assumed that trust will follow status, and therefore more precautions must be taken to see that the trust is not abused."

Any exposure of unethical procedures, submission to unnecessary hazards, deceit, or jury wiretapping in experimentation not only arouse fear, but also destroy trust. Whenever advantage is taken of the helplessness or unprotected state of the subject, whenever deceit is involved, trust is impaired. This rules out the use of stooges or other disguised participants. A very important obligation is that the scientist, supported as he is by society, maintain the trust given him.

Society and the Individual in Human Experimentation

In earlier years human experimentation proceeded with fewer hindrances than were accorded work on dogs, and from those free and easy days certain abuses emerged. In all the current charges and counter charges a clear issue can be seen emerging. It is above personalities; it is above legalistics; it is simply this: in experimentation in man, is the individual subject to get first consideration or does that consideration belong to society? It is time the debate was directed to this fundamental issue.

Society certainly has rights, recognized in law and by all men of good will, in the invasion of the individual's privacy by the census, in the legal requirement of certain standards of education and of hygiene, in the required reporting of venereal disease, in vaccination, in maintenance of civil order, in the required acceptance of the military draft (in wartime a life-or-death issue).

It is evident that at times society properly acts against the wishes of the individual, without his consent. Thus, while freedom of choice, of consent, must stand very high, the freedom is not total, as illustrated in the examples just mentioned. At times decision has to be made against the individual to protect society. This is a grave and central problem.

Notwithstanding these and other exceptions where society must come first, there are, it seems to me, cogent reasons why, *as a general principle*, the individual must have priority in human experimentation. We can examine these reasons in the hope that advocates for society's preeminent position will also tackle this complex problem and attempt to substantiate it from *their* point of view. A healthy society requires healthy treatment of individuals. A considerable debate, a truly divisive debate on this theme, has been going on, like an iceberg, seven-eighths below the surface, one-eighth above.

Unfortunately, those who opt for society—the most good for the most people, as they sometimes say in justification of their free-wheeling experimentation—have scornfully tagged those who believe in the supremacy of the individual as "zealots": "one-track zealots," "zealous crusaders," "extremists," and so on. The descent into name-calling is regrettable.

So far, those who choose "the greatest good for the greatest number" have had their derisive say. The other side has not chosen to reply in kind. But they could. Some labels harsher than "zealot" could be brought to bear on those who "for the most good for the most people" have injected live cancer cells without the recipient's knowledge; those who chose to withhold penicillin for "scientific" reasons from 525 young airmen with streptococcus throat infections when their own prior work had demonstrated the overwhelming effectiveness of the agent in preventing rheumatic fever, with the result that 25, according to the investigators (or 70 plus, according to a medical officer present) contracted rheumatic fever; on those doing thymectomies and skin grafts in babies for "scientific" reasons only; on those who have deliberately infected 250 mentally defective children with hepatitis virus; on those who deliberately risked and *repeatedly* demonstrated liver damage from a suspected toxic drug in children—in a center for mentally impaired and delinquent children; on those many experimenters on the human heart, where its integrity has been jeopardized (one experimentalist had 15 deaths in his first 150 cases); on the current repeated testicular biopsies in young prisoners—the list could be very long. What kind of a tag will the society they profess to cherish place on such investigators as these?

Curiously, the competence of anyone who dares to question the morality of such experiments as those just mentioned may be impugned, unless he is an expert in the field of cardiology, or immunology, or toxicology, or an authority on liver disease, or an endocrinologist, and so on. But it cannot be soundly maintained that questionable experimentation is rare.

In the hospital, decisions are constantly being made where some lives are saved and others lost. The control of these decisions is the issue and, where research is involved, it becomes particularly difficult to be certain of one's judgments. While society has a direct oversight of such decisions, through the hospital's committee on research and in its committee on ethics, such groups nevertheless usually place greater emphasis on safety for present lives than on the welfare of masses of future lives (society). The wish of the individual cannot be the controlling element in deciding which life will be saved, which lost. The interests of society, as well as the interests of the individual, must figure in this; the question is, Which should get first consideration? When it comes to research, the more official (societal) the risking of lives, the more important becomes the valid consent of the subject. He must not be pressed, coerced, or tricked into a collaboration he would reject if fully informed.

As Calabresi (9) has put it, we want a decision which reflects a societal choice and society's control when subjects are to be risked for the common good; but, at the same time, we do not want society to lose its role as protector of individual lives. These desires are conflicting; but both are essential to a decent society. In clinical investigation the physician has the power to determine which shall prevail at a given time; but an unanswered question is, Has he the right? A rigid and pedantic following of customs, rules, codes, and laws could easily lead to the untenable conclusion that the only supreme public interest is that of society. This conclusion is false: the individual has rights too, and *these*, barring a few exceptions, must predominate.

> Consent, though very useful in preserving the appearance that society hardly ever condones the sacrifice of an individual against his will, is unlikely to suffice where a too obvious societal choice to take victims is involved. . . . Even more important, consent cannot serve as the general control item which determines when the future good requires the taking of present lives. Therefore, it is to the development of a workable, but not too obvious, control system which can use various forms of consent as an adjunct that scholars seriously concerned with the problem of saving future lives and at the same time not undermining our commitment to the sanctity of individual present lives ought to be devoting themselves (9).

The extraordinary preoccupation of individuals and groups with "codes" seems to be an attempt to place upon society the responsibility for what may happen during human experimentation: if these "guides" are accepted by society and the individual experimenter has followed them, then, if an accident occurs, the responsibility is not the investigator's, at least not his alone, but society's. Man is not willing to take the responsibility for mankind in the mass, only for individuals; but, rather unfairly, he expects mankind—society—to protect him! One difficulty is that the individual experimenter cannot know how much risk society wants him to take for future benefit; but consultation with his peers can provide some help.

As mentioned, society is the protector of individuals; but society must also maintain control over situations which inevitably lead to sacrifice of some for the common good. Consider the decisions made during operation of the artificial kidney. The widow whose children are educated and grown will be rejected by society's committee in favor of the father of several young children. The widow will be allowed to die and the other saved by dialysis. It is more comfortable to look at this from a positive and general approach, to think that society has saved the young father rather than that it has sacrificed the widow; life has been sustained. The situation is different when specific lives are jeopardized or sacrificed, as in the numerous examples described (4), dealing with questionably ethical or unethical human experimentation with no immediate gain for a specific individual. Then the gain is for faceless mankind in the future and the bystander is disquieted.

There is some quiet opposition to respect for the patient's rights—more than a casual observer might suppose. Not long ago a distinguished scientist said to me, with some heat, "The individual is not infinitely valuable." This clashes with the view of Guttentag (15) and with my view: "the use of force is not justified on a single person, even if millions of other lives could be saved by such an act. [One realizes] the act would not just save millions of lives but that, as an amoral act from the standpoint of democratic brotherhood, it might create millions of amoral sequels, and that the moral history of mankind is more important that the scientific." The act also clashes with Reston's (27) view: "If there has been a decline of decency in the modern world and a revolt against law and fair dealing, it is precisely because of the decline in the belief in each man as something precious." Downgrading of the individual is common in attempts to justify unethical experimentation. An experiment does not become ethical post hoc: It is ethical at its inception or it is not.

"Statistical" Morality

At the Dartmouth Convocation on the great issues of conscience in modern medicine, Warren Weaver (31) described statistical morality as derived from the "prejudice against even permitting any one known specific individual to sacrifice his life for the common good," and yet, he continued, "we have to, in a great many circumstances, submit a lot of individuals to a partial risk," with the result that even though "the risk is only one in a million, when a million are involved, one man will be dead with our acquiescence. . . . It is a comfort to our conscience that we don't know *where* it occurred or *when* it occurred. But that individual is just as dead as though we knew all about it." In such deep waters we strive for balance, but sometimes emerge with little more than questions and tangled arguments.

For example, in discussing new and uncertain risk against probable benefit, Lord Adrian (1) spoke of the rise in Britain of mass radiography of the chest. Four and a half million examinations were made in 1957. It has been calculated that bone-marrow effects of the radiation might possibly have added as many as 20 cases of leukemia in that year; yet the examinations revealed 18,000 cases of pulmonary tuberculosis needing supervision, as well as thousands of other abnormalities. That 20 deaths should occur from leukemia was only a remote possibility, but, Lord Adrian asks, even if they were a certainty, would they have been too high a price to pay for the early detection of tuberculosis in 18,000 people?

One can see some fascinating similarities and equally fascinating differences when comparisons are made between the attitudes and goals of those whose concern is accident law, on the one hand, and those involved in human experimentation, on the other hand. Guido Calabresi (9) has made penetrating studies in this area. For example, the issue in medical experimentation is the risking of lives to save other lives, but almost always in accident law the issue is loss of life because prevention costs too much, or is too much trouble, or interferes with the pleasure of many. Here, once again, considerations of statistical morality are at hand: Calabresi points out that accidents at grade crossings cost a certain number of lives each year. These accidents could easily be prevented, as far as knowing what to do is concerned; but the cost of eliminating all such crossings is simply "too much." He points out that, too, automobiles cost 50,000 lives each year and most of these could doubtless be saved if slower and less transportation were accepted. However, the cost in terms of pleasure and profit would be "too high." Automobiles are driven on relatively cheap but also relatively dangerous tires. Other risky economies are effected until the missionary zeal of a Nader calls attention to the fact that the automobile is unsafe at any speed.

When the consideration is a faceless number in jeopardy, even if that number is known to be large, the matter is often treated with indifference; but if the situation involves a specific man trapped in a coal mine, no cost or effort is spared to rescue him, for "we know the man trapped in a coal mine, just as we often know the patient subjected to experimentation; the statistical accident victim we do not know—so we can ignore him" (9). Thoughtful people must have known for a long time that health and life are sometimes lost in medical experimentation, but very little was said publicly about the matter. It was only when twenty-two *specific*, sick, elderly Jews had live cancer cells injected into them without their knowledge and when, at about the same time, I, quite by coincidence presented a ten-year study of ethics in medical experimentation where *specific* examples were given, that a considerable public furor occurred (4, 7). No such result was present in the preceding decade when I not infrequently spoke and wrote in general terms on the same subject. The somewhat extreme reaction of praise by some and condemnation by others occurred only when I dealt with specific examples.

To return to Calabresi's analysis of the situation: there appears to be "a deep conflict between our fundamental need constantly to reaffirm our belief in the sanctity of life, and our practical placing of some values (including future lives) above an individual life." How can we resolve this conflict? Several factors must be incorporated into any satisfactory resolution. These can be suggested tentatively. Perhaps man is not very much interested in mankind in general; he cannot relate to many persons, but *can* identify with a single individual. Another, quite different, ingredient in any understanding of the problem surely is the fact that accidents are the result of chance, carelessness, or factors beyond control, whereas human experimentation involves risk deliberately taken.

When many accidents occur as a consequence of some particular situation, restrictive corrective law is hopefully applied, sometimes with such halfway measures as warning devices at grade crossings, rather than corrective elimination. But restrictive law has not yet been applied to human experimentation in any very comprehensive way. One of the few certainties in this complex field is that it *will* be, if certain abuses, such as those in the case material mentioned, are not soon corrected. It is probably always a mistake to invoke legal action in any rapidly changing situation, such as that found at present in human experimentation. Scientists and physicians may be able to correct practices that need correction before coercive and restrictive legislation is imposed.

Situation Ethics

My purpose is to examine a world where there are, basically, only two inhabitants; the investigator and his human subject. In this world there are a number of imponderables, not the least of which is "situation ethics," so eloquently described by Professor Joseph Fletcher (14). If I may be permitted an oversimplification, it is a world where circumstances alter cases, a pragmatic world where things are what their results are. I realize I can easily get myself into difficulties with the philosophers. Bertrand Russell has already likened the situation to a bath that heats up so imperceptibly one doesn't know when to scream. But let me give you one example from our world of experimentation, for we dare not overlook the relevance of the situation to the ethics thereof. Let me do this and I promise to scamper hastily off this thin ice.

When the wonders of penicillin were new, but recognized, and the supply heartbreakingly meager, a shipment finally arrived in North Africa in World War II. The hospital beds were overflowing with wounded men. Many had been wounded in battle; many had also been wounded in brothels. The problem: Which group would get the penicillin? By all that is just it would go to the heroes who had risked their lives and who were still in jeopardy, and some were dying. By all that is just these would get the penicillin. They did not, nor should they have. It was given to those wounded in brothels. Before indignation takes over, let us look at the situation: First, there were desperate shortages of manpower at the front. Second, those with broken bodies, broken bones, were not going to be swiftly restored to the battle line even with penicillin, whereas those with venereal disease, on being treated with penicillin, would in a matter of days free the beds they were occupying and return to the front. Third, no one is going to catch osteomyelitis from his neighbor; the man with venereal disease remains, until he is cured, a reservoir of infection and a constant threat. In terms of customary morality a great injustice was done; but I think not, in view of the circumstances. I hope you agree.

Ends and Means

Lasting progress in understanding the problems inherent in human experimentation can come only if one searches out the areas where men of good will differ, where sound principles seem to be in conflict. I have tried from time to time to identify these; for example, the conflict between the rights of the individual and the rights of society.

We have now a far more subtle confrontation—ends and means. A prevalent school of moralists declares that the end does not and will never justify the means. George Edward Moore disagrees categorically: "What I wish first to point out is that 'right' does and can mean nothing but 'cause of a good result,' and is thus identified with 'useful': whence it follows that the end always will justify the means, and that no action which is not justified by its results can be right," and this of course is pragmatism. It is also comforting to know that Lao-Tzu said long ago that true philosophy is like a pickle on the knee. I think I know what he meant—that it is difficult to keep a balance, that systems are prone to tumble. Where the experts can so easily harass each other is not safe territory for me, but, whereas I earlier thought that the end does not justify the means, Professor Fletcher (14) has since thoroughly convinced me that *only* the end justifies the means. I should like, therefore, to mention how my conversion came about, for the debate is most relevant to certain basic problems in human experimentation. I now propose to follow Professor Fletcher.

If the end does not justify the means, what does? And he answers,

"Nothing." Human experimentation without a definite purpose is meaningless—worse, it is unethical. Unless there is an end to serve, action is haphazard. ". . . means without ends are empty and ends without means are blind—it is the coexistence of its means and ends that puts it in the realm of ethics." This is no place for a universal: not any end will justify any means. Our concern is greater for the end than the means; but at the same time the means must be "appropriate" to the end. The means "ought to fit the end, ought to be fitting"; they are not neutral. In the situationist's circumstances-alter-cases view ". . . *ends*, like means, are relative . . . all ends and means are related to each other in a contributory hierarchy . . . *not only means but ends too are relative*, only extrinsically justifiable. They are good only if they happen to contribute to some other good than themselves."

The usual procedure of self-justification is to say that the progress of science "requires" the experimentation done on the uninformed, unconsenting patient. Or it is said by some medical editors that objection to publication of certain unethical studies "would block progress." These typical remarks have been voiced many times; so often, in fact, that one wonders where the medical schools have failed. Rarely are such remarks made by men who apparently could not care less about ethical failure. Far more often they are made by young and old who have simply failed to see clearly the issues involved, owing to failure to consider them.

It is often said that one lives in a materialistic age, in a materialistic world. A considerable number of individuals are in the unhappy and untenable position of accepting the results of unethical experimentation while disapproving the means.

If any further example were needed, atomic fission dramatically emphasized the inseparability of science and ethics. We can hardly separate the moral equivalents bound up in means and ends in this area; but we can, for example, take a pragmatic stand and say with Lord Russell that means are determined by science, whereas ends are set by desire. We can say with Kant that people must always be treated as ends, never as means alone.

This is "the scientist's ethic, and the poet's, and every creator's:

that the end for which we work exists and is judged only by the means which we use to reach it" (6).

At the end of his short life, nearly a hundred years ago, the mathematician and philosopher Clifford had this to say, "If I steal money from any person, there may be no harm done by the mere transfer of possession; he may not feel the loss, or it may even prevent him from using the money badly. But I cannot help doing this great wrong towards Man, that I make myself dishonest. What hurts society is not that it should lose its property, but that it should become a den of thieves; for then it must cease to be society. This is why we ought not to do evil that good may come; for at any rate this great evil has come, that we have done evil and are made wicked thereby" (6).

ACKNOWLEDGMENT: Much of the material in this chapter appeared originally in *Research and the Individual*, by Henry K. Beecher, M.D. (Little, Brown and Company, 1969), and is published with permission of Dr. Beecher and Little, Brown and Co.

REFERENCES

(1) Adrian, E. D. "Priorities in Medical Responsibility" (Jephcott Lecture). *Proc. Roy. Soc. Med.* 56 (1963): 523–528.

(2) Beecher, H. K. "The Powerful Placebo." *J.A.M.A.* 159 (1955): 1602–1606.

(3) Beecher, H. K. "Evidence for Increased Effectiveness of Placebos with Increased Stress." *Amer. J. Physiol.* 187 (1956): 163–169.

(4) Beecher, H. K. "Ethics and Clinical Research." *New Engl. J. Med.* 274 (1966b): 1354–1360.

(5) Beecher, H. K. "Consent in Clinical Experimentation: Myth and Reality" (editorial). *J.A.M.A.* 195 (1966): 34–35.

(6) Bronowski, J. *Science and Human Values.* New York: Harper and Row, 1965.

(7) Brook Lodge Conference. Symposium for Science Writers sponsored by the Upjohn Company, Kalamazoo, Michigan, March 22, 1965.

(8) Cahn, E. "Limits for Experimentation" (excerpt from "The Lawyer as Scientist and Scoundrel: Reflections on Francis Bacon's Quadricentennial"). *N.Y. Univ. Law Rev.* 36 (1961): 1–12.

(9) Calabresi, G. "Reflections on Medical Experimentation on Humans." Conference on Ethical Aspects of Experimentation on Human Subjects at the American Academy of Arts and Sciences, Boston, Mass., November 3–4, 1967.

(10) Cooley, T. M. *A Treatise on the Law of Torts.* 2nd edition. Chicago: Callaghan, 1888.

(11) Crime Commission, President's, 1967. *The Challenge of Crime in a Free Society. A Report by the President's Commission on Law Enforcement and Administration of Justice.* Washington, D.C.: Gov't. Printing Office, 1967.

(12) Editorial, *New York Times*, June 8, 1968.

(13) Ernst, M. L., and A. U. Schwartz. *Privacy: The Right to Be Let Alone.* London and New York: Macmillan, 1962.

(14) Fletcher, J. *Situation Ethics.* Philadelphia: The Westminster Press, 1966.

(15) Guttentag, O. E. "The Problem of Experimentation on Human

Beings. 2. The Physician's Point of View." *Science* 117 (1953): 207–210.

(16) Ivy, A. C. "The History and Ethics of the Use of Human Subjects in Medical Experiments." *Science* 108 (1948): 1–5.

(17) Lasagna, L., and H. K. Beecher. "The Optimal Dose of Morphine." *J. A. M. A.* 156 (1954): 230–234.

(18) Lerner, D. In Ruebhausen and Brim, *Columbia Law Rev.* 65 (1965): 1185 (footnote 1).

(19) Liberman, R. "An Experimental Study of the Placebo Response under Three Different Situations of Pain." *J. Psychiat. Rec.* 2 (1967): 233–246.

(20) Mead, M. "The Human Study of Human Beings." *Science* 133 (Jan. 20, 1961): 163.

(21) Mead, M. "Ethical Aspects of Experimentation on Human Subjects: From the Standpoint of Anthropology." Conference on Ethical Aspects of Experimentation on Human Subjects at the American Academy of Arts and Sciences, Boston, Mass., November 3–4, 1967.

(22) Mead, M. "Research with Human Beings—a Model Derived from Anthropological Field Practice." Conference on Ethical Aspects of Experimentation on Human Subjects at the American Academy of Arts and Sciences, Boston, Mass., September 26–28, 1968; *Daedalus* 98 (1969): 361–386.

(23) Modell, W. "The Primary Ethical Decision" (editorial). *Med. Trib.* (May 24, 1967), 11.

(24) Moore, George E. *Principia Ethica*, p. 146. Quoted by J. Fletcher, in *Situation Ethics*. Philadelphia: The Westminster Press, 1966.

(25) Platt, Lord Robert. "The Ethical Basis of Medical Science." *Sci. Basis Med. Ann. Rev.* (1966).

(26) "Privacy and Behavioral Research. Preliminary Summary of the Report of the Panel on Privacy and Behavioral Research." Panel under chairmanship of Kenneth E. Clark, Dean, College of Arts and Sciences, University of Rochester; *Science* 155 (1967): 535–538; also *American Psychologist* 22 (1967): 345–349.

(27) Reston, J. "Washington: The Capital and the Easter Story." *New York Times*, April 18, 1965.

(28) Shils, E. A. "Social Inquiry and the Autonomy of the Individual." In *The Human Meaning of the Social Sciences*, Ed. D. Lerner. New York: Meridian Books, 1959.

(29) Starzl, T. E. In "Transplantation: Existing Legal Restraints," D. W. Louisell. Discussion of, in *Ethics in Medical Progress*. Ciba Foundation Symposium. Boston: Little, Brown, 1966.

(30) Warren, S. D., and L. D. Brandeis. "The Right to Privacy." *Harv. Law Rev.* 4 (1890): 193–220.

(31) Weaver, W. "The Problem of Statistical Morality." The Dartmouth Convocation of Great Issues of Conscience in Modern Medicine, Sept. 8, 9, 10, 1960; *Dartmouth Alumni Magazine Suppl.* Nov., 1960.

INDEX